CW01003901

COSMOPOLITAN'S

# HEALTH
# & BEAUTY
# HANDBOOK

# ZEST

COSMOPOLITAN'S

# HEALTH
# & BEAUTY
# HANDBOOK

# ZEST

Edited by
CHRISSIE PAINELL

Written by
PATTIE BARRON
NICKY LYON-MARIS
ESME NEWTON-DUNN
CHRISSIE PAINELL
VERITY SMART
SOPHIE VINCENZI

EBURY PRESS • LONDON

*To my father, John, and to Russ*

Published by Ebury Press
Division of The National Magazine Company Ltd
Colquhoun House
27–37 Broadwick Street
London W1V 1FR

First impression 1988
Copyright © 1988 The National Magazine Company Ltd
Illustrations Copyright © 1988 Penny Sobr

ISBN 0 85223 644 1 (Hardback)
0 85223 649 2 (Paperback)

Editor Miren Lopategui
Designer Bill Mason
Illustrator Penny Sobr
Picture Researcher Joan Tinney

Typeset in England by Chapterhouse Typesetting Ltd., Formby, L37 3PX
Printed and bound in Italy by New Interlitho, S.p.a., Milan

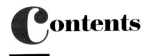

# Contents

# how to use this book

Welcome to Cosmopolitan's Zest, a health and beauty handbook that brings you the latest advice and tips in a fun-to-read, season-by-season format.

You can dip in and out of the sections, quickly and easily: a new heading introduces a new subject, which may be just a few paragraphs in length or may run over several pages. Continuation headings appear in the top left-hand corner of the pages.

A special note: there are many great workouts throughout the book. However, before you start an exercise programme for the first time, or try a movement that is new to you, please do read the feature Body Wisdom and Exercise Essentials on pages 18–23, particularly the pre-exercise programme checklist on page 19.

If you are in any doubt about your ability to do any of the exercises, or if you are worried about your health, check with your doctor. None of the information in this book is intended to replace medical advice given to you by your general practitioner or a specialist.

Enjoy using the book and try to put a little time aside for yourself each week to exercise, to relax, and to pamper yourself. You'll soon see the big beauty and well-being benefits!

# ZEST SPRING

A new season, a fresh start. On the following pages, the secrets of looking sensational. Discover the difference exercise can make to your energy levels. Follow our stress-beating strategies. Create sleek body contours *fast* with our weights workout and take a look at the best hip and thigh treatments around. Let's go!

# body sculpting

Strength training doesn't mean you have to start pumping iron, or that you'll wind up with bulky muscles. Whichever body contouring method you choose – calisthenics, free weights, or a gym machine system such as Nautilus or Universal – you can reap these big beauty benefits:

\* improved muscle tone and quick changes in body shape

\* improved muscle endurance and muscle power

\* good posture

\* prevention of muscle imbalances which can lead to injuries

\* quick improvement in specific problem areas such as thighs, stomach, upper arms.

Read on for the pros and cons of each method and essential weight training info:

*Calisthenics are exercises which stretch and tone muscles without using any equipment – for instance, press-ups and sit-ups.* **Fitness pluses**: *they can be done wherever you have space to move your arms and legs freely. Weight-bearing exercise helps prevent osteoporosis. The body toning exercises in the Swimsuit Shape-Up Plan (page 25) are an easy and effective way to tone your body from top to toe in a few minutes each day.*

Free weights. Working out with free weights combines calisthenics and weight-lifting with dumb-bells or barbells to strengthen specific muscle groups. A good programme will include warm-up and cool-down stretching exercises. **Fitness pluses**: there are big shape-up benefits and quick results that you can see – muscles look toned and firmed and you can measure inch-loss. You can reduce fat but could gain weight since muscle is heavier than fat.

Warning note: Training too hard and with too much weight may cause injury, so start slowly and be cautious. Instruction is vital when working out with barbells.

*Weight machines work on the principle of varying resistance. The safest and most efficient are designed to work the muscle at optimum resistance through the range of movement. You need a gym near you with a fairly complete set of machines and on-hand instructors to check that you are using the equipment correctly, and to set you targets.* **Fitness pluses:** *as with free weights, you see improvements in muscle tone, and progress in the amount of weight lifted. This method is safer than using free weights because the machine, and not you, holds the weights and your body position is stabilized.* ►

## WORKING-OUT WITH WEIGHTS: VITAL KNOW-HOW

✳ Rule of thumb: Performing more repetitions, quicker, with lighter weights gives muscle endurance and tone. Heavy weights (which you can only lift up to a max of 6 reps.) lifted slowly build strength and muscle bulk, although it is very hard for women to reach body builder bulk.

✳ It is important that you don't use the same muscles two days running. When muscles are worked, the tissue breaks down and repairs during rest periods to become stronger than before. Lift something or stretch too far before the muscles have recovered properly and you're risking injury to these weak points. If you want to work out every day, you should alternate upper, mid and lower body workouts to give muscles time to repair in between.

✳ Always warm up with large body movements – arm circles and brisk walking – followed with stretching.

✳ Use control when lifting/pushing, or pulling weights, and move more slowly, not faster, to work muscles thoroughly. When you speed up you use momentum, not muscle. Don't jerk movements.

✳ Don't let your mind wander – it's important to concentrate on using the correct muscles in order to isolate them, otherwise you could be 'cheating' on the exercise and using the wrong muscle groups, or could get hurt by letting the weight 'fly' or drop.

✳ Remember to breathe – never hold your breath or tense up. Focus on exhaling on exertion.

✳ Never leap on to a new-to-you weights system, even if you are familiar with other brands of gym equipment. The machines may work on a different principle – hydraulic instead of cam, for instance – and may require different body positioning and muscle action.

✳ Whichever system you choose, make sure you're using the equipment to maximum advantage. If using a cam system, for example, check that the joint of the area to be worked out – hip, knee, elbow – lines up with the centre of the cam (the machine's point of rotation) for better – and safer – strength pay-offs.

✳ Never lock joints while lifting.

✳ Pause only momentarily between repetitions to keep the muscles contracted and working.

✳ Ideally, you should stretch after each machine routine while the muscle group you've been working is warm.

✳ Don't add ankle weights to legs during aerobic activities (walking, jogging, cycling, aerobic dance classes) as they can strain the lower back and joints.

✳ Don't get so caught up with weight training (if you are results-motivated it's easy to do) that you forget that increasing stamina (cardio-vascular workouts with aerobic exercise) and flexibility are integral parts of the fitness equation.

✳ Do muscle-strengthening calisthenics, such as push-ups, leg lifts, etc., and weight training at the end of a workout or on a day when you're not involved in your main aerobic exercise. Otherwise you will build up the 'oxygen debt' and may be too exhausted at the start of your workout to get the biggest benefits from the endurance activity (advises Dr Kenneth Cooper of the Institute for Aerobics Research, Dallas, USA.)

**W**arning note: *One problem with some systems is that weights progress in large increments of 2.2 kg (5 lb) or 4.5 kg (10 lb) which may cause injuries in women. Take care that you don't try to lift too much too soon. Some women are too small to use some machines.*

---

## WHAT EXERCISING REGULARLY DOES FOR YOU

✳ Exercise improves the quality of your sleep (but don't schedule an aerobics session just before bedtime).

✳ Exercise helps control poor eating habits. Regular exercisers are more likely to eat healthily and drink water not coffee; inactive people tend to head for junk food and alcohol.

✳ Exercise does great things for the skin.

✳ Exercise curbs high blood pressure and reduces heart disease risk.

✳ Exercise helps you relax and is mood-boosting. Working out encourages the production of beta-endorphins, hormones produced by the pituitary gland in the brain which fight stress and deliver a good feeling.

✳ Exercise improves the absorption of nutrients in the body.

✳ Exercise is proven to be a contributory factor in preventing osteoporosis (brittleness of the bones.)

✳ Exercise keeps your weight stable. And it burns calories.

✳ Expending energy gives you more energy!

✳ Oh, and exercise gives you the best-looking body of your life!

---

# the lightweight workout

**T**his workout is designed for those with a reasonable level of fitness. If you haven't exercised recently, reduce the weight and/or number of repetitions. Work at the repetitions indicated for 3 workout days, allowing the muscles to recover for a day in between, then increase the repetitions by five. If you want to do more, increase the repetitions rather than the weight, to avoid bulky muscles. Use dumb-

bells of 1–1.3 kg (2½–3 lb). Ankle weights around 900 g (2 lb).

---

*Remember, when working out with weights, perform the movements very slowly – work the resistance, don't swing in and out. If you suffer from a lot of neck and shoulder tension, weights could add to this. Stretch out and relax neck and shoulders beforehand.* ►

**11**

**SPRING**

# ZEST

Note: When doing the upper body exercises, check your posture to prevent putting strain on the back. Keep knees slightly bent, stomach pulled in, tilt the pelvis and tuck the buttocks under. Warm up your before you start this workout by Bridget Woods of The Fitness Centre.

**OUTER THIGH:** Lie on side, stretched out along the floor. Roll hip forwards and stretch leg out to side as you slowly lift and lower. Keep knee facing forwards. Repetitions: 20 each leg. ▼

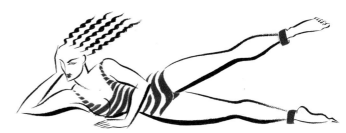

**UPPER ARMS AND SHOULDERS:** Check your body alignment, ensuring knees are bent and bottom tucked under. With arms stretched out in front at shoulder-level and shoulder-width apart, alternately bring weights up to shoulder. Don't drop elbows but keep shoulders relaxed and down. Repetitions: 10 sets. ▼

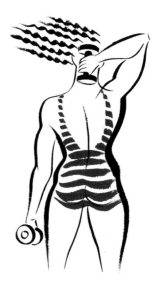

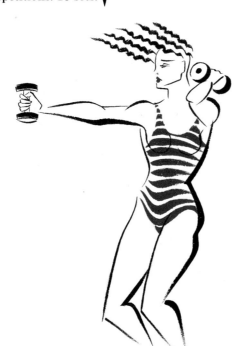

**TRICEPS:** Stand with feet hip-width apart, knees bent. Stretch right arm up, keeping opposite shoulder down. Slowly lower weight, keeping elbow pointing up. Repetitions: 10 each side. ▲

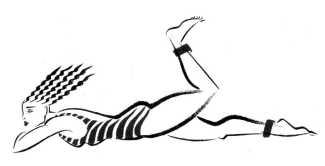

INNER THIGH: Lie with lower back stretched out. Bend back leg and keep hip pressed forwards. Lift other leg, keeping the inner thigh facing ceiling. To check you're working the correct area, press down on inner thigh with fingers – the muscles should feel contracted. Repetitions: 20 each leg. ▼

BUTTOCKS AND BACKS OF THIGHS: Stretch out along the floor, resting chin on hands. Bend knee, flex foot, and, keeping hip bone on floor, press ball of foot up to ceiling. Slowly lower to floor, keeping leg bent; repeat, remembering to keep body lengthened. Repetitions: 20 each leg. ▲

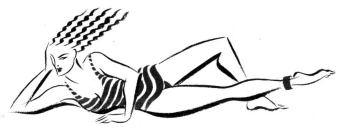

BICEPS: Check body alignment. Keep elbows into waist (this helps control) and shoulders down. Alternately raise and lower dumbbells slowly (don't extend the arms fully). Repetitions: 20 each side. ◄

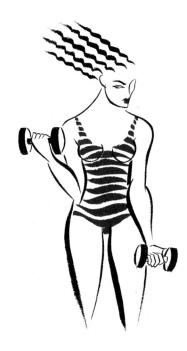

*You don't have to knock yourself out to build a strong body! These easy moves firm, sculpt and strengthen.*

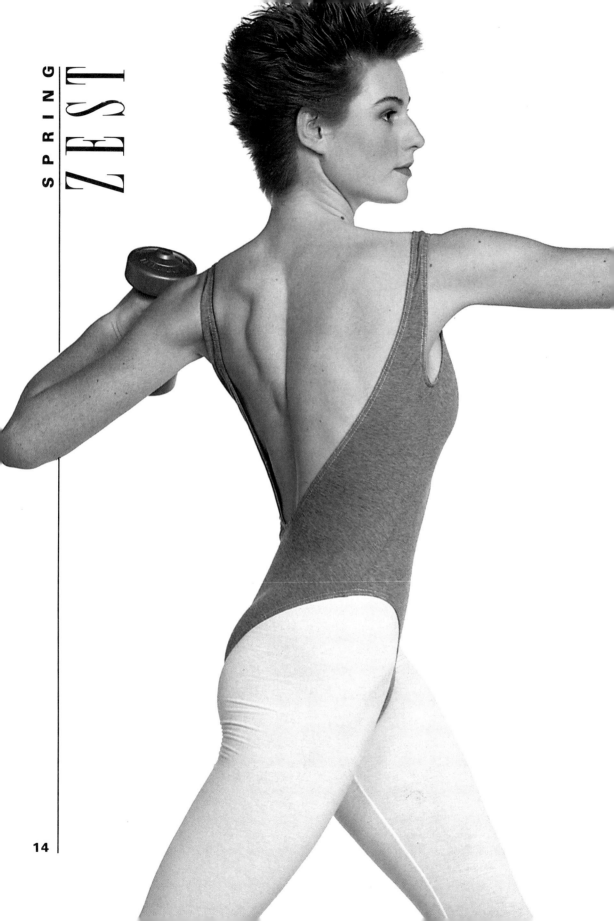

# ZEST

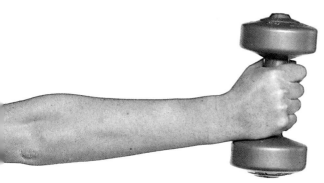
Lightweight workout continued

## HOW TO STICK WITH IT

**F**ind an exercise programme that suits your personality, as well as your fitness needs. If you want a creative, more mind-directed workout look to martial arts, yoga, or Pilates. If you are results-oriented, try calisthenics, free or fixed weights. For competitive types, sport is the obvious answer.

———

*In a study of over 10,000 women and men, the University of Michigan, USA, found that 'inner directed' or self-motivated people exercised much more regularly than those classified as 'outer-directed' (those more likely to stick to patterns set by others). These traits were a stronger force than age, education or income brackets.*

———

**T**ry to stick with a regular programme for at least 6 weeks. Dr Kenneth Cooper of the Institute for Aerobics Research, Dallas, believes that it takes this long to make the habit stick. You'll then begin to notice such a change in your physical and emotional well-being that you'll probably be ready to commit yourself for life.

———

*Don't launch from nil into a complete programme – the enthusiasm that originally fired you can quickly peter out and injuries and boredom set in. Build up from 10 minutes instead.*

———

**D**on't diet and exercise at the same time when you start an exercise programme, advises sports physiologist and coach Angela

UPPER BODY (works arms, shoulders, chest and back): Stand with feet hip-width apart and stomach pulled in. Twist from waist, bending right leg, and press forward with opposite arm. Take arm back. Repeat on other side. You can do this with arms at any height: the higher the arms, the stronger the workout. Repetitions: 20 each side.

**15** ▶

Cannell. 'Many women decide to totally change their lifestyle and throw their body into total confusion. They feel exhausted and decide it's not working for them.'

---

*If you get bored fast, divide up your aerobic workout. For instance, do 10 minutes on the stationary bike, then run on a treadmill, use a stair climb or skip. Remember that aerobic exercise must be continuous to be effective and that you mustn't stop completely while you are training.*

---

'**O**ne-on-one' workouts with personal trainers are a growing trend in gyms. They individualize your programme, motivate you and help you gain maximum benefits safely in minimum time. Trainers even call you up if you don't show for a workout! Joining a gym is a good motivator whether or not they have one-on-one. The instructor/supervisor will devise your workout regime and check your progress regularly. There are now many workout machines that feature electronic feedback, showing you how many miles you've clocked up, and the number of calories burned; high-tech rowing machines even have VDU screens so that you can 'race' a competitor. Recently introduced, there are now fixed weight machines that 'talk' to you, coaxing you on!

---

*Setting goals is a great motivator – provided they are realistic. Take regular fitness tests at your health club, aim to move on to advanced classes, to take up circuit training or train towards playing a sport.*

# **d**e-stress stretches

These easy stretching exercises can be done at the desk or when you arrive home, to revitalize you after a tough day. Warm your body up before you do the exercises. Before each stretch take a deep breath in, and then let out a long, sighing breath as you relax.

***WAIST AND SPINE STRETCH***: *Standing, centre your pelvis. Rest hands on shoulders, lengthen spine and rotate torso to right keeping body straight. Hold for 30 seconds, breathing normally, and repeat to left. A broomstick placed across the shoulders adds leverage and helps keep spine lengthened.*

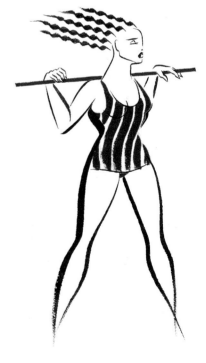

## EXERCISE – HOW TO FIND THE TIME

* Make exercise top priority. Recognize the importance of making it a habit – sporadic exercise doesn't strengthen your body because there is no training effect. Look at it in the same light as everyday routines like healthy eating, cleaning your teeth, getting enough sleep.

* Exercise first thing in the morning – it's the only way to make sure it becomes part of your day! Plus you'll start the working day with a sense of achievement. Research has found that exercising in the morning burns the same number of calories as in the afternoon – *but* a.m. activity uses one-third more calories from fat deposits. Set the alarm clock now!

* If you are considering investing in home exercise equipment, a rowing machine will give the best results. Rowing tones, firms and conditions your whole body and improves your heart/lung fitness. Unlike cycling or running, rowing works all major and most minor muscle groups in the back, stomach, arms, shoulders and legs.

* Invest in dumb-bells and use the weights workout on pages 11–15 to increase your strength. Buy an at-home exercise video with aerobic and stretching exercises. Don't just launch in – remember to allow time for warm-ups and cool-downs.

* Walk everywhere; don't take the lift or escalator – climb the stairs!

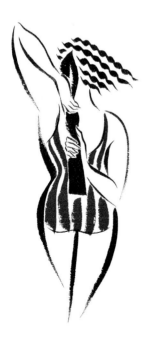

*Ten minutes exercise a day is more beneficial than an hour a week, advises expert Esme Newton-Dunn.*

**SHOULDER STRETCH**: *Bend left arm behind back, working hand up towards right shoulder. Place right hand behind shoulder and try to bring hands together, hold for 30 seconds. If hands won't meet, hold a small towel and work hands gradually towards each other. Repeat with other arm.*

A desk job can mean an eight-hour circulation slow-down. Try these fast-to-do exercises.

Dancer and personal trainer Clayton Marshall suggests this exercise for the legs: Sit in a chair which supports the back. With left foot flat on floor, raise right leg parallel to floor, knee locked. Bend raised leg slightly 5–7.5 cm (2–3 inches) then straighten again. Complete 10 times and repeat with other leg. Terrific for strengthening front of thigh muscles and problem knees.

Esme recommends this circulation rev-up for lower extremities: Stand on the edge of a step and lift and lower heels to strengthen and stretch calf muscles. If you don't have a step, simply rise up on to balls of feet several times and then bend forward from knees, feet flat on floor, for the counter-stretch. Flexing and pointing feet also works.

Keep your shoulders and neck relaxed by repeating these movements frequently during the day: Lift both shoulders up towards ears and circle firmly back, squeezing shoulder blades together. Repeat at least 5 times. Next, sitting upright, tilt head to right, circle to centre and then around to the left. Repeat in opposite direction. Don't roll head back – it puts strain on the neck.

# body wisdom & exercise essentials

So you want to be fit and healthy? You want to develop a sleek and trouble-free body so that you can look and feel great for the rest of your life. You determine that you will start your new regime *this* Monday.

By Wednesday you are aching, stiff and hungry, and reading an article which tells you that exercise causes injuries and that being fit doesn't mean you're healthy anyway. Confused and disillusioned, you give up!

This is a sad but frequent tale. When the big aerobics boom arrived from the USA, there weren't enough teachers to satisfy the growing demand for classes. For most people, aerobics was the Deep End. Totally unprepared bodies were hurtled through a rigorous routine with little or no supervision. *Watch the supple body at the front bend and twist effortlessly while you follow as best you can with creaking joints and tight muscles.* No wonder there were injuries! But now we have professional associations for teachers and improved training.

But having a properly qualified

# PRE-EXERCISE PROGRAMME CHECKLIST

✳ Do you smoke?

✳ Do you have high blood pressure?

✳ Do you have a high level of fats in your blood? (If you've had a blood test you may have been told this – otherwise, don't worry about this question.)

✳ Do you take regular exercise?

✳ Is your life sedentary?

✳ Is there a history of heart disease, heart murmurs or strokes in your close family?

✳ Do you tend to be overweight?

✳ Do you suffer from stress?

✳ Are you taking any medication?

✳ Do you suffer from asthma, diabetes, or any other condition?

---

teacher is only half the story. Before you embark on an exercise programme, you should develop your own body awareness which tells you when to go on – and when to stop.

Ask yourself the basic pre-exercise questions (above).

If you feel healthy, are under 35 and have answered 'no' to most of the above questions, there's no need to consult your doctor before taking up an exercise programme. If, however, you have answered 'yes' to three or more of the first 8 questions, then exercise could affect your heart. Obviously, if you are taking any kind of medication this might also affect you while exercising, so check with your doctor. Similarly, if you are pregnant, suffering from asthma, diabetes, have had recent surgery or have

back or joint problems, check with your doctor about which programme would suit you best. If you suffer from a medical condition, please also inform your instructor before exercising.

## HOW FIT DO YOU NEED TO BE AND WHERE SHOULD YOU START?

Most people associate fitness with stamina-type exercises – should you jog a mile or run a marathon? But the question you should really ask yourself is, What do you want to be fit *for*? There's no point in maintaining an athletic level of fitness unless you participate in a sport. Your level of fitness should relate to your lifestyle, otherwise you'll find it difficult to maintain. Find something you enjoy doing, therefore, and vary your exercise as much as possible to avoid becoming bored.

*The basis of all effective exercise is good posture. Many people develop postural problems – through their occupation, constantly carrying a heavy bag, or emotional stresses such as stooping because of being*

*Your level of fitness should relate to your lifestyle, otherwise you'll find it difficult to maintain.*

self-consciously tall. If you have developed bad postural habits, your body may be out of alignment and you will put strain on muscles, ligaments and joints if you exercise. Work on your posture while looking in a mirror. If, like many women, you tend to stand with your lower back over-arched, you will find that when you line yourself up straight in the mirror, you feel very unnatural. In this case it is important to unlearn your old habits. The same will apply to new exercises. Well taught body conditioning classes are therefore the best place to start an exercise programme – and to keep up good postural control.

If you have problems with your back, hips, knees or ankles, ensure that the aerobic exercise you choose will not jar these joints. Instead of high-impact aerobic dance or jogging, try a mini-trampoline or low-impact aerobics such as walking briskly or swimming.

## MAXIMUM EFFECT, MINIMUM STRAIN

Always start in a beginners' class. This will give you time to develop the correct technique for each exercise at a pace you can cope with. Try to understand each exercise so that you know:

∗ Which muscle group you are trying to work and what this will achieve.

∗ Where you should feel the exercise and the correct position to achieve it.

∗ How to adapt the exercise

should you have difficulty in performing it.

There is both a hard and an easy way to perform any exercise. As most of us are not pre-selected to the athletic elite, we each have to adapt our own strengths and weaknesses to the exercise routine. Remember to train, not strain!

## TIME WELL SPENT

The most important point to bear in mind is that you should exercise regularly. Once a week is just not enough for any real benefit because you will lose the training effect. Twice a week is really the minimum – this could consist of one session of swimming and a class or a brisk walk. Three to four sessions a week is ideal, alternating the days you exercise to allow the body time to recover. More than four sessions a week, however, is counter-productive and unnecessary.

To improve your stamina you will need to build up to at least 20 minutes of aerobic exercise in each session. You can usually build up your stamina quite quickly, unless you are extremely unfit. But your joints, muscles and ligaments will not be able to adapt so quickly to the new demands you put on them. This applies less to swimming and brisk walking than to running, as these activities impose much less stress on the joints. Above all, check that your exercise programme contains all the elements of the fitness equation: stamina, stretch (for flexibility) and strength.

**The warm-up:** Before beginning any kind of vigorous exercise you should always warm up your muscles to prevent strain. This should include some general stretches (see pages 158–161) and movement to gradually raise your pulse rate and body temperature. Your muscles and connective tissue will be nourished by the increased circulation and will become more supple. Remember this when you're going for a jog round the block or before a game of squash, as well as in aerobics classes.

**The essential cool-down:** After energetic exercise, it is all-important to slow your pulse rate gradually. Don't suddenly stand still, sit or come to a halt at a red light – keep walking or jogging on the spot. Never skip the cool-down or you could become dizzy.

If you take time away from your normal exercise you should always start from the beginning and not from where you left off. If you're reasonably fit, it shouldn't take long to train up to main-tenance level again.

# a erobic exercise

Aerobic energy is defined as energy produced in the presence of oxygen. Aerobic exercise improves your cardio-vascular (heart/lung) performance and your stamina. Thus, steadily building up your training level will increase your level of aerobic fitness. Exercise expert Esme Newton-Dunn explains: 'Unless you stimulate your body to increase its ability to take in, pump and utilize its oxygenated blood, the whole system is going to remain weak and sluggish and your energy levels will be down, making even simple everyday tasks a drudge.'

When exercising aerobically, it's important to monitor your heart rate regularly. Heart rate is measured as pulse rate, and as a rule the fitter you are the lower this will be. Begin by finding your resting pulse rate. (Ideally, this should be done first thing in the morning when you are relaxed.)

Measure the rate by placing three fingers above the centre of the inside of your wrist and counting the number of beats per minute (b.p.m.) with the help of a wrist watch. The average resting pulse rate in a woman is 72 b.p.m., though there may be considerable variations on either side. Use the resting pulse rate to gauge your fit-ness. Take your pulse rate repeatedly after exercising – the quicker it returns to its resting

*It is important to monitor both your pulse and how you feel when exercising. You should feel comfortably out of breath while exercising aerobically.*

rate (and the lower the resting pulse rate becomes) the fitter you will be. If you are unfit and your resting pulse is high, even quite gentle exertion can raise your heart rate.

To calculate your target heart rate during aerobic exercise, subtract your age from 220 and then multiply by the training level required, usually 65% to 80% of that figure.

e.g. $220 - 20 = 200 \times \dfrac{65}{100} = 130$ b.p.m.

### New-think aerobics

*Recent studies have shown that working out at lower training rates of 40% to 60% is still beneficial. Exercising at a lower intensity is better for joints and muscles because you reduce the chance of damage – low-impact aerobic dance takes out the hops, so one foot is always on the floor, making it less frenetic and more enjoyable for most people. You will, however, need to exercise for longer to gain the same benefits.*

### Aerobics: The weight-loss workout

Aerobic exercise is the most effective way of controlling your fat levels, provided, of course, it is combined with a long-term healthy eating plan. The bonus with the aerobic workout is that you can raise your metabolic rate – and it stays high after exercise. Recent research has shown that fat-burning benefits are longer-lasting than originally believed. The fat-burning mechanism is believed to come into play after about 30 minutes of sustained exercise – a big plus point for low-impact aerobics. High-impact aerobics should not be performed for longer than 30 minutes or there may be a risk of musculo-skeletal injuries. High-impact aerobics include running, jogging, orienteering, dancing and skipping. Walking, swimming, cycling, cross-country skiing, canoeing, circuit training, skating and rowing are all low-impact aerobic workouts.

*Note:* It has recently become popular to put weights on the body when running or taking an aerobics class as a means of increasing the intensity of the workout and of conditioning the upper body. Beware, however, of using hand or wrist weights if you suspect you have any cardiovascular problems.

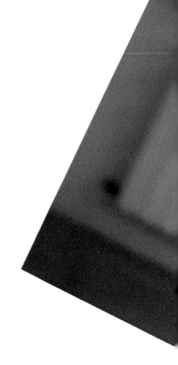

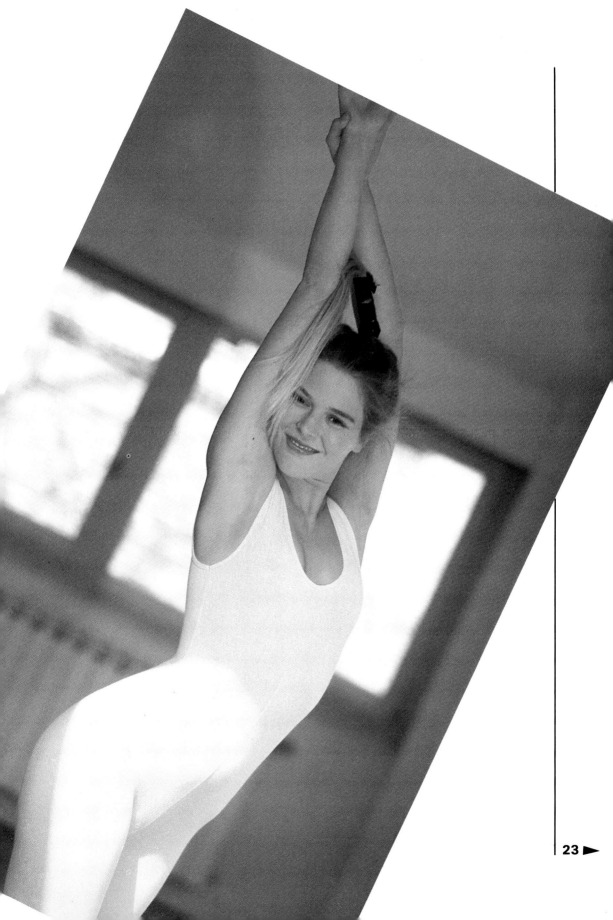

# Skipping: the fitness scoop

Skipping gives you a great cardio-vascular workout on the spot. As one gym trainer points out, 'Sports people skip to improve their game but it's a good method of building fitness on its own, improving posture, co-ordination, agility, speed, flexibility as well as stamina. Body areas that most benefit: shoulders, legs and buttocks.

### EASY-GOING STYLE

*Always skip on a soft surface (not concrete) and wear aerobic shoes. Because skipping involves hopping as well as stepping, don't take it up if you have joint weaknesses in your legs or Achilles tendon problems. Keep your back straight, head up and breathe properly. Movements should be small and neat – small jumps, turning the rope mostly with the wrists.*

*If you're unfit, spend a few weeks walking and jogging before you start your programme. Warm up thoroughly to avoid straining the body, by walking around the room for a couple of minutes, then do some gentle stretches. Concentrate particularly on the Achilles tendon: face the wall, lean on hands, right leg bent and left leg straight out behind you. Push heel gently towards ground.*

### PICK UP THE PACE

Start at a pace of 2 jumps a second (120 a minute) and work up to 3 or 4 a second. High knee raises put extra emphasis on the front of thighs and calves. Turning the rope backwards is good for toning the bust. Slowly build up to three sessions of 15 or more minutes a week, with rest days in between.

*A good rope helps your style:* choose one with ball bearings, preferably leather. The length should be twice the distance from your shoulder to the ground when holding the rope out at arm's length.

## ANAEROBIC EXERCISE

Anaerobic energy is produced without the presence of oxygen. It is of high intensity and usually brief duration. Anaerobic exercise builds your sprint speed – helps you run for the bus, for instance. Most anaerobic sports will involve some aerobic exercise as well.

Sports which use anaerobically generated energy include racquet sports such as squash and tennis, baseball, softball, football, badminton, basketball, cricket and hockey.

Anaerobic exercise is not as effective for weight loss as aerobic exercise because most of the energy is drawn from stores of glycogen in the muscles which are quickly replaced.

# Swimsuit shape-up plan

Want to get into shape in time for summer? Sleek body contours are only a few minutes away with our simple, no-sweat workout. The programme strengthens and firms the body's tough-to-tone spots – waist, chest, arms, stomach, buttocks and thighs – and has been designed to alternate between upper, middle and lower body zones so that each area has two days' rest in between.

Begin each sequence with a brisk walk around the room for 2–4 minutes, swinging your arms, to warm your whole body up, then do the specific warm-up and

*Hit the beach toned from top to toe with our super-effective 5 minutes a day exercise plan*

stretch given for each area. Make sure all movements are performed smoothly and do not cause pain (stop if they do). Advance by repeating the sequence. If you're in reasonable shape, but need to firm up wobble-prone zones, you can expect real results within 4 weeks.

**MONDAY AND THURSDAY: UPPER BODY WORKOUT**
Before and after each session, circle shoulders forwards and backwards. Circle each arm slowly backwards 8 times.

UPPER BACK: Standing, grasp hands behind you at lower back. Keeping elbows bent, squeeze your shoulder blades and upper back together and then release. Repetitions: 10–20.

BACKS OF ARMS: Rest hands behind you on a stable chair, with feet hip-width apart and parallel, and knees bent. Raise and lower body using arms only, keeping shoulders down. Repetitions: 10–20. ►

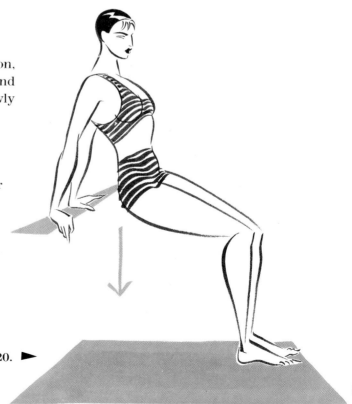

**SPRING ZEST**

CHEST: Easy press-ups – kneel down and lean forward to rest weight on straight arms. Raise legs and cross feet behind you, keeping tummy in and shoulders down. Lower and raise body by bending and straightening arms, keeping your back straight. Repetitions: 10–20. ▼

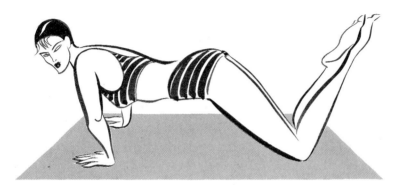

BICEP CURL: Holding a light weight (approx 675 g (1½ lb)) stretch arm out to the side at shoulder height. Slowly lift and lower weight, keeping your shoulders down and elbows up. Repetitions: 10–20.

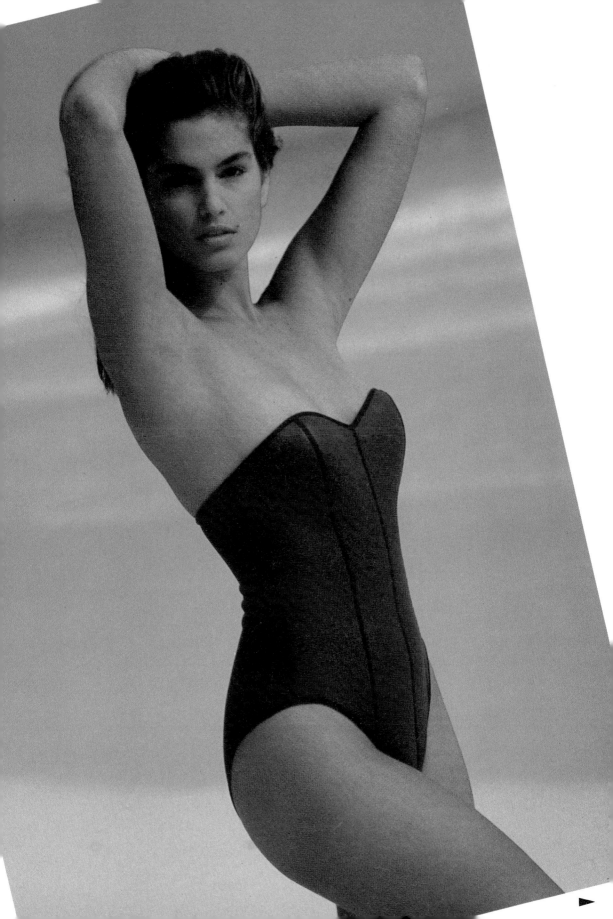

SPRING *ZEST*

## TUESDAY AND FRIDAY: MID-BODY WORKOUT

Before you begin, lie on your back with knees bent and tilt your pelvis backwards so stomach pulls in, pubic bone tilts up and lower back presses on to the floor. Pull in as hard as you can for a slow count of 4, breathing out. Breathe in as you release muscles slowly. Repeat several times. When you've finished the sequence, draw knees up to chest and gently squeeze.

WAIST: To work right side – roll on to your left side. Keeping your body straight, prop head up on hand and place right hand in front to steady you. Lift both legs up to side. Repeat on left side. Repetitions: 5–10.

STOMACH:

1. Lying on your back, bring knees up to chest, cross ankles and then semi-straighten legs. Curl head and shoulders up and draw pubic bone towards you, lifting your tailbone slightly. Make sure that your stomach pulls in and down. Half uncurl and repeat. Repetitions: 10. ▶

BUTTOCKS:

1. Lie on your back, thighs parallel and feet hip-width apart, with stomach pulled in. Lift bottom and squeeze buttocks together. Repetitions: 20–40.

2. Turn your legs and feet outwards (with knees over feet); lift and squeeze outer butttocks. Repetitions: 20–40.

3. With feet, knees and thighs together, lift and squeeze. (Works inner buttocks.) Repetitions: 20–40. ▼

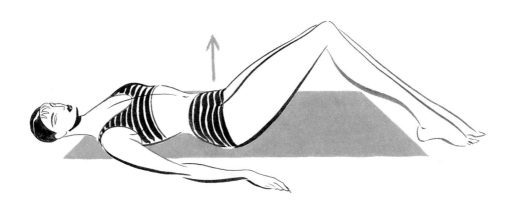

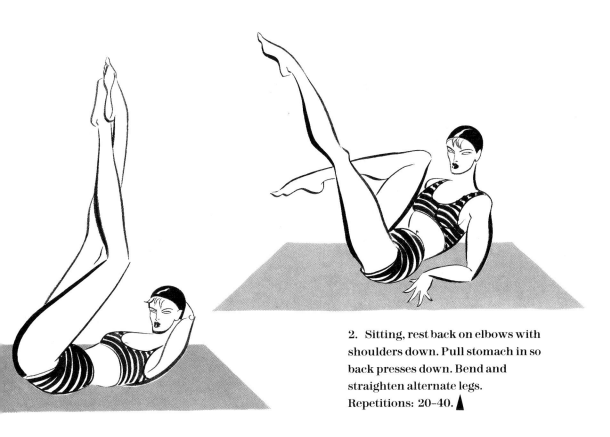

2. Sitting, rest back on elbows with shoulders down. Pull stomach in so back presses down. Bend and straighten alternate legs. Repetitions: 20–40. ▲

---

## WEDNESDAY AND SATURDAY: LOWER BODY WORKOUT

A specific warm-up isn't necessary for the lower body. The initial brisk walk will have warmed up your muscles sufficiently.

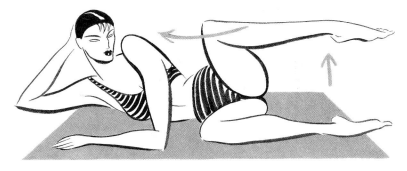

OUTER THIGH: Lie on right side and bend both knees to hip level. Pull in tummy to flatten back and roll top hip and shoulder forward.

Open and close legs keeping lower leg on floor. Repetitions 20–40. Straighten leg to advance, 10–20 repetitions. Repeat on other side.

SPRING ZEST

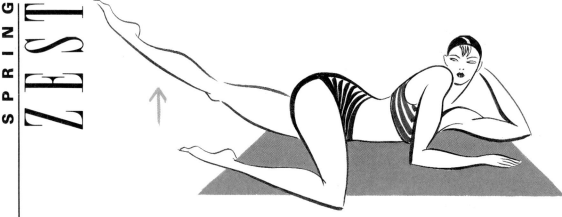

INNER THIGH: Drop right knee in front of body. Straighten underneath (left) leg. Flex foot and lift and lower underneath leg, exercising the inner thigh muscles. 20 repetitions. Repeat on other side.

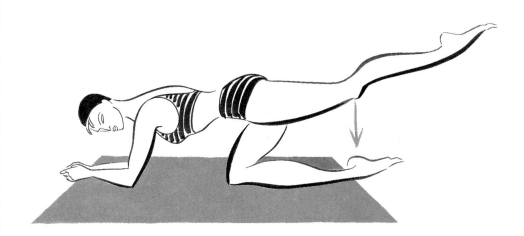

BACK OF THIGHS: Kneel down and rest weight between knees and forearms. Hold stomach in, and straighten leg behind. Make small, smooth lifts, keeping hip down. Repeat with other leg. Repetitions: 20–40 each leg. ▲

STRETCH FOR BACK OF THIGHS: Lying down, place left foot on the floor, knee bent and draw right knee towards chest. Gradually straighten leg out as far as possible, keeping thigh on chest. If this is easy, straighten out left leg as well. Hold stretch for at least 30 seconds. Repeat exercise with left leg.

# hip and thigh shapers

If lumpy skin on hips and thighs is a familiar problem, you won't care that the medical profession largely denies the existence of what beauty experts term cellulite. Cellulite is due to compartmentalization of fat with excess fluid, and restriction of the capillaries which carry blood to the area. The excess fluid seeps between the cells making the skin look puffy. Over the years, fibrils of collagen (connective tissue proteins that contribute to the skin's plumpness and suppleness) wrap round the fat cells, restricting capillaries. The result is nodules, which can be felt as bumps under the skin. You don't have to be fat to have cellulite – any body size can be cellulite-prone – it is an inherited beauty spoiler which can also affect the knees and stomach and will not be shifted by dieting.

*An action plan to help beat cellulite can include:*

* *A sensible healthy eating plan, plus lots of water, to help eliminate toxins.*

* *A regular workout programme that you feel you can really keep to.*

* *Deep-down massage to stimulate circulation and help break down fatty deposits.*

* *Body contouring products.*

* *Salon/spa treatments.*

*Get ready for summer with these skin and body contour seekers.*

## TOXIN-FREE EATING

Adopt an eating programme which is as free as possible from toxins, ie unnecessary preservatives and additives which contribute to the build-up of toxic waste and excess fluid. Cut down on salt, which is high in sodium – a major culprit in fluid retention. Potassium helps displace sodium so eat plenty of potassium-rich foods such as potatoes, spinach, bananas, beans and fruit juices, to counteract the effects of salt. Grapes and fresh pineapple are believed to enhance the breakdown of fats.

Smoking is one of the worst offenders in affecting the tone and texture of hips and thighs. Nicotine impairs the absorption of vitamins essential for the skin's health; carbon monoxide, carried to the skin surface by normal circulation of blood, constricts the capillaries that feed the tissues. Smoking also speeds up the breakdown of collagen, which is essential for maintaining elasticity and firmness.

### THE EXERCISE CONNECTION

*An exercise programme boosts circulation, feeding skin cells with oxygen and eliminating waste. All forms of exercise will be beneficial but anything aerobic is especially good. Work to strengthen the often neglected inner thigh. Avoid, however, building lots of muscle over long-established cellulite, but break down the cellulite first with massage.*

### THE MASSAGE MOVEMENT

Use the power of massage. It is essential in stimulating circulation and de-toxifying the skin's structure. Normally, the body's toxins are carried out of the body by lymph, but if you're very tense, lymphatic drainage can be restricted by tight, knotted muscles, resulting in toxin build-up. Massaging with an aromatic oil, such as neroli to relax the nervous system, can help in two ways: by de-tensing muscles so lymph fluid can flow freely, and by restoring good posture. When massaging, work upwards towards the heart using sweeping movements.

**Massage mitts:** Brushing the skin with sisal mitts increases circulation and sloughs away dead surface cells so that body contouring products can penetrate more effectively. Massage tools with rubber nodules or rollers soften collagen fibres and encourage fat to disperse.

### BODY CONTOURING PRODUCTS

*Body contouring products can help speed results, when used in conjunction with the other cellulite-beating factors described above. There are now products produced for both long-established and more recently formed, easier-to-treat cellulite. All contain ingredients which help to break down cellulite and tone and firm the skin, such as seaweeds, vitamin E, and plant extracts such as ivy, butcher's broom and horse chestnut.*

## THE SALON SOLUTION

**In** beauty salons and health farms, heavy-duty help is at hand. Ultrasound, thalassotherapy (powerful jets of warm, mineral-laden sea water are directed at the dimpled areas), lymphatic drainage with pressotherapy (inflatable rubber 'stockings' mechanically pumped to increase the flow of lymph), Ionithermie (see below), massage and injections are available – all are expensive, may require a course of treatments and are sometimes painful. All good salons will recommend exercise and an anti-cellulite eating plan in addition to treatment.

**G5 massage** using a series of electric hand-held gyrating heads is an effective cellulite beater. The salon may begin with a paraffin wax treatment to stimulate circulation, then follow up with G5 and manual massage.

**Ionithermie** is a treatment that gives instant results – you'll feel motivated into making the effort to exercise and eat well to maintain and improve the impressive inch-reduction that Ionithermie produces.

Treatment areas are measured (waist and thighs to the knees for cellulite), then ampoules and creams formulated to break down fatty tissue, speed circulation and firm tissues are applied one by one while you lie on a plastic mattress. A clay is smoothed on next and electrodes inserted in between the layers to conduct galvanic current (to increase absorption of the products) and faradic current (to 'passively' exercise the muscles). You feel a tingling sensation in your muscles and the current is stepped up to a level you find comfortable. Half an hour later, the hardened clay is removed in one piece, any creams left on the surface are wiped off and the body is measured. A total loss over the area of 7.5 to 37.5 cm (3–15 inches) is usual. Clients are advised not to shower or bath for 6–8 hours because the creams are still active.

---

Make a habit of cleansing, toning and moisturizing your body as you do your face. Silken, supple skin needs to be worked at daily to refine texture and restore elasticity. Dead cells on the skin's surface can block pores and make skin appear dull and flaky. Exfoliating with a friction mitt, loofah or a gentle body scrub will help ensure that the freshest, newest skin is always exposed, stimulate circulation and increase cell turnover. Never slough until you irritate the skin, or abrade inflamed or infected areas.

If you're counting down to a holiday in the sun, use sloughing treatments all over and blitz spotty backs with once-a-week purifying masks as part of your pre-sun preparations. When using exfoliating products, rinse skin very thoroughly, as traces left on the skin can irritate.

Body skin on the legs and arms tends to be particularly dry because there are fewer oil glands. Skin needs moisture: the key to keeping it soft and supple is sealing in the moisture that's already present. So use a light oil or body lotion while skin is still damp to form a protective film over the surface.

---

**33**

# What's best for breasts

✳ Hot baths and showers are bad news for bust-conscious girls. Use cool water to stimulate circulation.

✳ Never go on 'crash' or very low calorie diets – as well as being potentially very dangerous to your health, they lead to loss of muscle and cause stretch-marks.

✳ The firming effects claimed for bust creams are disputed by doctors and dermatologists but do keep the skin soft and supple. Be very delicate when massaging breasts to avoid damaging the fibrous tissue.

✳ Pack a sports bra if you're off for a few days' holiday. The fresh air and scene-change could inspire you to go for a jog, join in a game of tennis or a spur-of-the-moment horse-ride. Never do any body conditioning without support: your bust has enough difficulty coping with gravity and bust tissue loses its elasticity for good. There is some evidence to show that running without adequate support can contribute to non-malignant lumps.

✳ Breasts are a sensitive area, so don't risk sunburn. Topless bathing calls for a high factor sunscreen on breasts and a total block on the nipples. Shower off salty or chlorinated water after swimming.

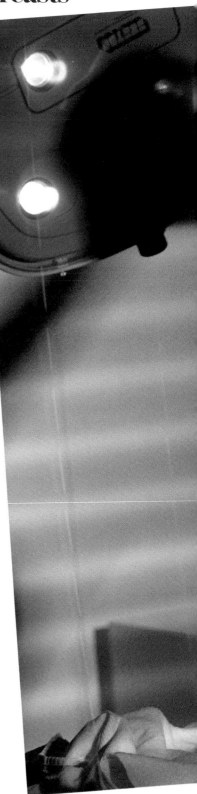

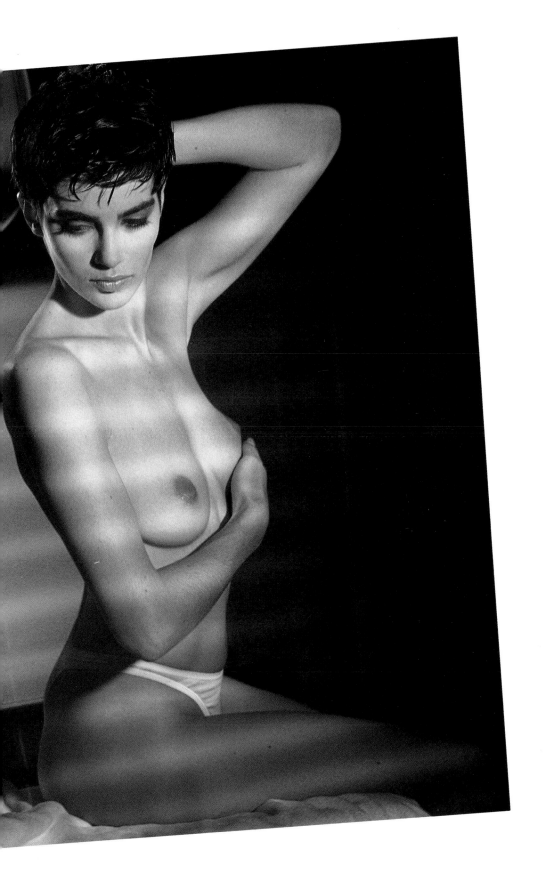

* Posture is the key to shape. Teenagers are often embarassed by body changes and many women believe their breasts are too small or too large: as a result they round their shoulders, which can lead to back problems later on. Yoga, body conditioning, ballet, Pilates (an exercise system that uses small lifting and stretching movements to tone the body) and the Alexander Technique are all terrific for correcting postural problems.

* Because breasts don't contain any muscle you can't firm or enlarge them with exercise, but you can strengthen the pectoral muscles at the sides and underneath to create a lifting effect. Try swimming as part of your exercise programme – breaststroke and backstroke are best for toning the pectorals. Arm movements in body conditioning/aerobics classes also boost pectorals. Whenever you have a free moment, try this exercise: cross your arms across your chest and hold the lower arms with the opposite hands. Press, as if trying to prise arms apart, relax, press. Check in a mirror – you should see your breasts lift when you tense.

* Thousands of women have breast augmentation operations each year. Surgery can also reduce breast size and rescue a drooping bustline. Operations should never be undertaken lightly – there is always a chance of complications, including the risk of increased difficulty in discovering breast lumps.

# health action: cystitis

Cystitis is a painful infection of the bladder, usually caused by bacteria. It can recur frequently and it is sometimes difficult to treat.

## Symptoms
When cystitis strikes, you will feel the need to urinate often even when there is no urine to pass and when you do urinate there may be burning pains, your urine may be cloudy and sometimes contain a little blood. You may also have a raised temperature and pain in the lower abdomen.

## Causes:
* *The female urethra (which leads from the bladder to the outside of your body) is only 2.5–3.7 cm (1–1½ inches) in length, whereas in men it measures about 20 cm (8 inches). Cystitis is therefore much more common in women. Germs from the anus can easily reach the urethra and bladder. Sexual intercourse can force bacteria up to the bladder. Perfumed or foaming bath products, antibacterial soaps, or vaginal deodorants may be responsible for recurrent cystitis. Washing powders, contraceptive sheaths and spermicidal*

# PREVENTIVE BREAST CARE

Most important breast info of all: from puberty every woman should take 5 minutes every month to check her breasts for lumps or any other irregularities in size, shape or skin surface. One in 15 women will develop breast cancer. Do the examination on the same day each month, 3 to 4 days after your period, when any hormonal changes will have normalized, and in the morning if possible, so that if you do find something unusual you can make an appointment immediately. If you are rushed for time, however, wait until you are relaxed and can make a thorough examination. Only one in 10 lumps is cancerous and many other breast changes can be caused by the contraceptive pill, pregnancy, etc.

A professional examination is recommended once a year and a mammograph (low-dose X-ray which can detect changes the hand can't feel) approximately every 2 years, but not be done under age 35.

*Monthly breast examination*

1. Lie on the bed, with a small folded towel under the shoulder of the side you are checking. With the arm of the breast you are examining raised behind your head to make any lumps easier to feel, place the other hand in the armpit and slowly trace your fingers down along the edges of the breast, gently but firmly.

2. Use the flat of your hand to push each part of the breast against the rib cage.

3. Using your fingertips, repeat this movement, moving in a circular direction, feeling for any alterations in shape or texture of the tissues. Around 40% of women have lumpy breasts – cystic swellings or bumpy areas – and need to know which bumps are 'normal' and harmless. When in doubt, consult your doctor or family planning clinic.

4. Examine your breasts in the mirror, looking for any dimpling or changes in texture and checking that the nipples look symmetrical.

---

*creams can cause allergies which may lead to cystitis. Stress can trigger an attack. Spicy foods or strong drinks cause cystitis in some people.*

### Precautions:

* *Always wipe from the front to back when you go to the lavatory and wash the area twice a day with plain water.*

* *Empty your bladder as soon as you feel the need to urinate.*

* *Both you and your partner should wash carefully before intercourse.*

* *Bruising during intercourse can trigger off the condition –hence the term 'honeymoon cystitis'. If your vagina is dry, use a bland lubricant and ask your partner to be gentle.*

* *If possible, pass urine after intercourse to flush away any bacteria.*

* *You may be more at risk just before your period, during pregnancy or menopause.*

### Treatment:

* *Drink as much water as you can to flush out the infection, from the*

*moment it starts, to prevent the urine becoming concentrated.*

✳ *Take a teaspoon of bicarbonate of soda dissolved in a little water to decrease the acidity of the urine and ease the burning sensation.*

✳ *Lie or sit down with hot water bottles against your lower back and lower abdomen.*

✳ *Drink herbal teas – juniper berry, marshmallow, parsley and comfrey. But don't drink regular tea, coffee or fruit juices.*

✳ *Take 1g of vitamin C every 6–8 hours to help alter the acid balance of the urine.*

✳ *There are over-the-counter remedies which may prove effective. (Remember to check the contra-indications on the packet – the preparation may not be suitable if you are pregnant, for example.) If symptoms persist, consult your doctor who will send a urine specimen to be tested for the organism responsible. Antibiotics may then be prescribed. Often there is no evidence of infection but the symptoms persist. Recurring cystitis or urinary infections can indicate a prolapse. When in doubt consult your doctor.*

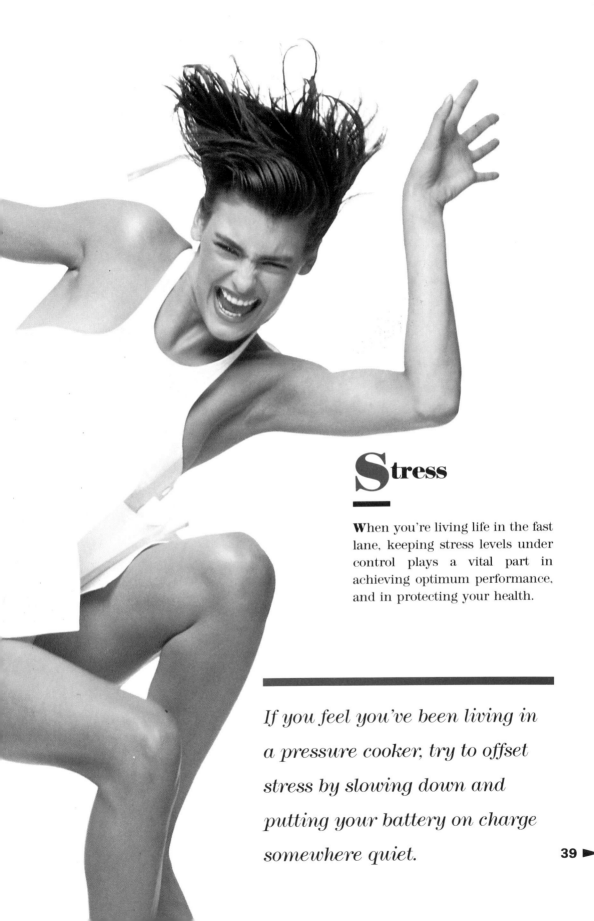

# Stress

**W**hen you're living life in the fast lane, keeping stress levels under control plays a vital part in achieving optimum performance, and in protecting your health.

*If you feel you've been living in a pressure cooker, try to offset stress by slowing down and putting your battery on charge somewhere quiet.*

Dr Malcolm Carruthers, Director of the Positive Health Centre, Harley Street, London, shows you the sure signs of stress, pinpoints personality traits and recommends strategies to reduce your stress load.

### IS STRESS TAKING ITS TOLL?

*Recognize the common mental and physical stress signals:*

* *Fatigue, anxiety and irritability, tension headaches, difficulty in sleeping.*

* *Skin under stress looks pale and is prone to frequent breakouts of spots. Stress is strongly linked to adult acne.*

* *Lack of enjoyment in home and work life.*

* *Undereating, overeating, or unhealthy eating – all of which deplete your energy levels. Undereating can lead to irregular heartbeats and mineral imbalances. One study at Cornell University, New York, showed that the more hours a woman worked and the more money she made, the more fatty foods she was likely to eat. Coffee, alcohol and drugs are serious health-squelchers that some of us turn to.*

* *Loss of sexual desire (one of the first things to go under stress).*

* *Nervous reflexes – particularly touching the hair, nose or ears; tooth-grinding or jaw-clenching; lip-biting or nail-biting; picking at facial skin or the skin around the nails.*

* *Outbursts and over-reactions.*

* *An inability to make everyday decisions.*

* *Stress-related ailments such as asthma, back pain, headaches, digestive disorders, skin disorders such as hand eczema, herpes.*

* *Hair loss. Doctors and trichologists are seeing an increase in the number of stress-related hair-loss problems in women. This may be related to the androgen hormone upsets in the system.*

### STRESS-BEATING STRATEGIES

* Keep as much rhythm and regularity in your life as possible. Your body is cyclical and doesn't like too much change. Eat regularly and go to bed/wake up at the same time each day. If you can't go to bed at the same time each night, still get up at the regular time the next morning.

* Vitamin C is used at a faster rate during periods of stress. Check you are eating fresh fruit and vegetables and consider taking vitamin supplements.

* Take regular stress breaks as preventive health care. If you feel you've been living in a pressure cooker, try to offset it by slowing

*Treat stress like income tax and do a regular audit.*

# STRESS AND PERSONALITY

Personality and behaviour patterns are leading protagonists in shaping reactions to stress and the ability to cope under pressure. We all display characteristics of predominantly one of two personality profiles, termed by psychologists as Type A or Type B.

There is a never-ending torrent of scientific data indicating that the stress-prone 'Type A' personality is at a far greater risk of heart attack, ulcers, hypertension, digestive disorders, diabetes, muscle aches and fatigue than the calmer Type B. As it is now recognized that 70% of all disease is stress-related, it's vital that Type As learn how to modify their behaviour.

Do you suffer from 'hurry sickness'? Leave important work until the last moment? Allow insufficient time to get to work and to appointments? Try to do two or more things at the same time? Eat as you work? Find it difficult to wind down on holiday? If so, you may be a Type A personality.

*Other Type A characteristics:*
Impatience; ambitiousness; competitiveness; aggression; a tendency to work hard; talking too fast or too loud.

Most people tend to be a mixture of the two – with a preponderance of one over the other, making them, say, Type A rather than Type B.

Type A women are more vulnerable than men to the subsequent detrimental effects on health: Type A men are 2 to 3 times more prone to heart attacks than Type Bs, whereas Type A women have a 4 to 5 times increased risk. Type As are more susceptible to fatigue and even have more accidents than Type Bs, who show the opposite of the above traits and are calm, easy-going and relaxed.

*Modifying Type A behaviour*
Follow the advice below – particularly important for Type As:
Try to leave your work at work.
Give yourself time to do things and do one thing at a time.
Take time off for rest and recreation – schedule it into your diary; you will work more efficiently between times.
Think of things worth being rather than doing, suggests Dr Ray Roserman.
Find a suitable relaxation method.
Make all these part of your lifestyle and you'll reduce your heart attack risks.

down and putting your battery on charge somewhere quiet.

✳ Treat stress like income tax and do a stress audit. Keep track of where your stress pressures are coming from – work, finance, relationships – and slow up in one area when you can.

✳ If you are feeling anxious and tense, count down slowly from 20.

✳ Become aware of what triggers a stress response. Take one day to monitor your reactions to events: what makes your heart beat faster, makes you clench your jaw, the palms of your hands go sweaty? Some health centres have biofeedback or chemofeedback machines which help you identify stressors. You are asked a series of questions and can see your physical, mental (and chemical) responses on a computer.

Stress continued

✳ Invest in learning a relaxation technique, such as meditation, yoga, Autogenics. These are all skills and will therefore need a good, well-qualified teacher.

✳ Relaxation tapes that feature a soothing voice talking you through progressive body relaxation have proven stress-reducing benefits. Find a voice you enjoy listening to – some of us prefer a female voice, others male.

✳ Exercise is instrumental in controlling stress. Aerobic exercise produces beta-endorphins – chemicals which will give your spirits a lift and boost your confidence.

✳ Eat a well-balanced, healthy diet. Limit your caffeine and sugar intake, and increase the amount of fresh fruit and vegetables that you eat.

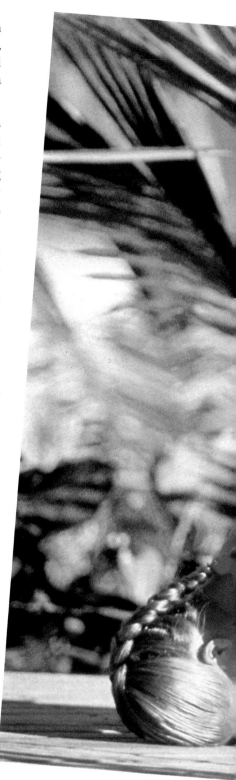

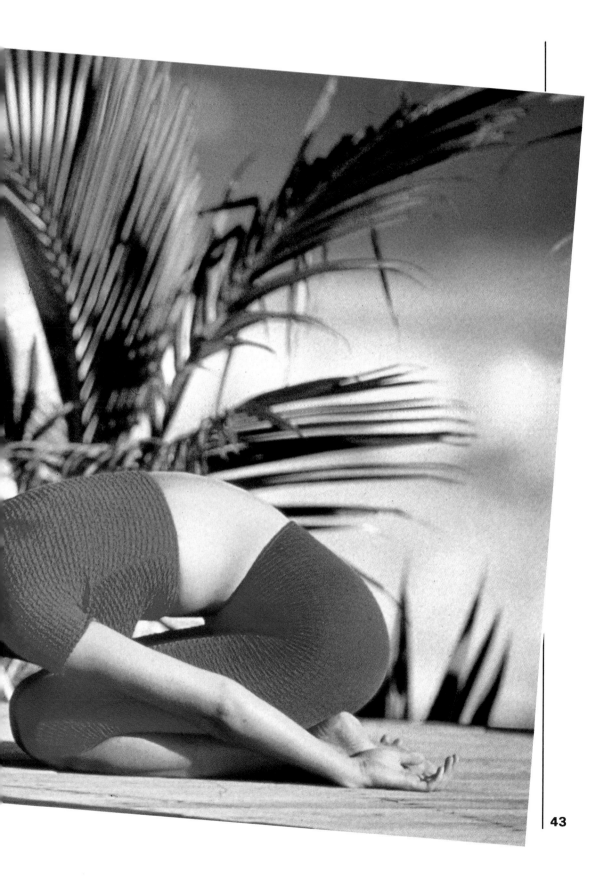

# ZEST SUMMER

Breezy and beautiful ... leap into this summer section and come up with bare-body poise. You can look sun-sational *and* save your skin. Investigate what outdoor sports can do for your body. Check the essential travel kit checklist. Beat the heat and indulge in delicious, healthy cocktails. You'll sail through summer in all-time great shape!

# Summer sun and sensitivity

Prickly heat affects 10% of the population. It causes skin to become inflamed and form tiny papules and once you have it, heat of any kind – even layers of clothes – will aggravate it. *Treatment*: apply cool compresses to the affected areas, pat dry and sprinkle on talc. Restrict ultraviolet exposure, especially avoiding the midday sun, rippling water or white surfaces, which reflect UV rays. Use a sunscreen with a high SPF. Avoid sweating.

*Waxing and shaving hair around the bikini line should be done at least 24 hours before hitting the beach, as sun, salt or chlorine can easily irritate.*

It's unlikely, but the cause of that itchy red rash you got lying in the sun could be caused by a reaction to the ingredients in your sunscreen. *Treatment*: stop using the product at once and apply cold compresses followed by calamine lotion. If you have sensitive skin, make sure you take adequate allergy-tested sun protection away with you.

Any skin type, not just sensitive skins, can suffer from photosensitization, where the skin reacts to the sun in the presence of plant juices, drugs or chemicals. Culprits you should avoid if possible when under the sun include medications containing diuretics, tranquillizers, perfume and aftershave, antibacterial soaps, and artificial sweeteners. Even if you've been exposed to sunlight for some while, an extra strong dose could tip the balance. *Treatment*: immediately soothe redness, itching or blistering with cold compresses, pool dips and showers and calamine lotion.

*White patches on the skin caused by a fungus (pityriasis versicolour) can increase after sunbathing. Preparations containing coconut oil may contribute to the problem, as this contains lauric acid which kills bacteria that normally might prevent fungus taking hold.* Treatment: *The patches will fade in time. Avoiding coconut oil products in future should help. A special shampoo can be used on the body (but not on the face).*

If you get sunburned – and you should of course know better and take every prevention against this – drink lots of cold water to counteract dehydration and cool your overheated system, and soak in a tepid bath. Pat on a lotion formulated to soothe sunburnt skin or pat natural yogurt or cucumber slices on to affected areas. Steer clear of the sun until the skin has completely healed. If burns are severe or the skin is broken, seek medical help.

**Heat exhaustion:** There are 3 types (all of which can be fatal). Symptoms of water-deficiency heat exhaustion include thirst, dry mouth and a rising temperature. *Preventive measures*: drink 6 cups of water in addition to the 8–10 you're advised to drink for summer well-being (6–8 is the general guideline in winter). Sip steadily through the day whether you feel thirsty or not. Thirst is not a good guide of dehydration.

*Treatment*: Rest in cool surroundings and drink half a litre of water every 15 minutes for 2 hours. Heat exhaustion due to salt-deficiency occurs if you have been sweating heavily during the first few days of acclimatization and not eaten properly due to a poor appetite. Fatigue, giddiness and severe cramps are indicators. Anhidrotic heat exhaustion is a rare sweat gland malfunction which occurs in people who have been in a hot climate for several months. *Treatment*: Rest in the cool with a high intake of salted drinks. Keep your body cool with frequent dips – bringing down your body and skin temperature periodically keeps your sweat glands from having to do all the work. Don't sleep.

*Keep your body cool with frequent dips – bringing down your body and skin temperature*

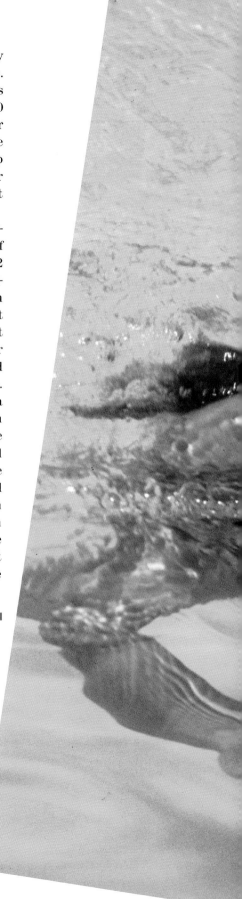

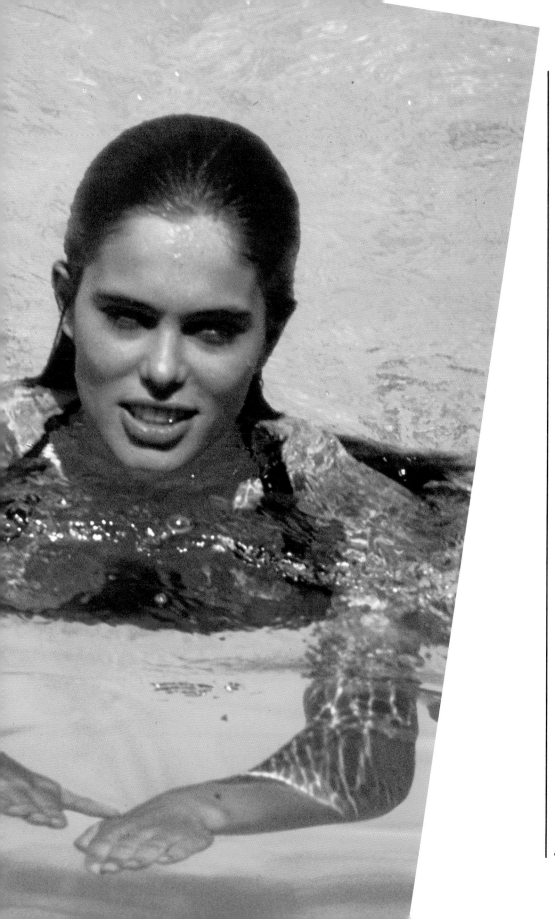

*If you begin to feel woozy or head-achey (and your skin may feel cool, clammy or very sweaty) retreat from the heat immediately. Cool your system with cold compresses, a tepid bath and sip liquids. Drink orange juice to replace lost* potassium. Add a proprietary salt and sugar solution and drink lots of water and juice with added sugar and/or salt. And lie down with your feet up.

If you don't feel better in 30 minutes or suddenly feel worse – become faint or disorientated, have headaches, stagger or start to convulse – call an ambulance or ask someone to drive you to the emergency department of a nearby hospital. With heatstroke (sunstroke is an incorrect term – you can get it without being in the sun), there is no sweating and the body temperature rises. In severe cases death can occur 2–4 hours after symptoms start. If someone you are with is affected, cool them down by removing their clothing and laying a damp towel on their body, hands and forehead to stop evaporation. Keep fanning them and spray cool water over them while waiting for medical help.

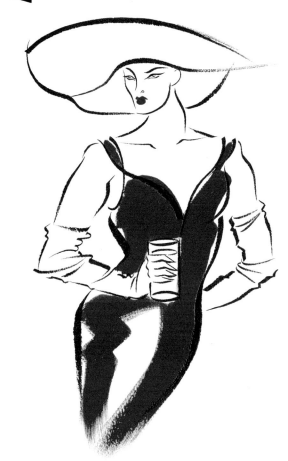

*If you begin to feel woozy or headachey (and your skin may feel cool, clammy or very sweaty) retreat from the heat immediately.*

# Cool exercise

When it's hot and humid, or maybe just one of those energy-sapping days, you need to adapt your fitness regime. Dehydration, heat exhaustion, heat cramps (which occur in muscle groups being used most) or heatstroke are among the less attractive by-products of working out the wrong way when the temperature soars. (There's also sunburn, skin chafing, prickly heat and discomfort!)

**The key to successful summer workouts:** keeping the body's core temperature at its usual comfortable level of 37.5°C (98.4°F). Overheating can be dangerous, even fatal. As you exercise, your body generates heat and needs to find a way to release it – that's when the usually efficient cooling system steps into play. Nerves are activated to send messages to your sweat glands. Minute muscles around the sweat glands contract so that perspiration is pumped out on to the surface of the skin. Meanwhile, blood rises towards the surface of your skin, where the cooled skin lowers the temperature of the blood and creates a cooling cycle. The danger begins when the cooling process is prevented from working properly.

**Choose safe summer sports-gear:** *Don't wear anything that stops you from perspiring. Choose clothes that are lightweight, loose, open-weave and in natural fibres, minimal and, ideally, white.*

*You don't want to let up on exercising just because the sun's on overtime. Follow these all-important stay-cool strategies for those days when the heat is on!*

**Don't overdo things:** *This is particularly important on hot, humid days, when the air cannot absorb the extra moisture your skin generates causing the sweat to roll off your skin in tiny, unevaporated globules. No evaporation, no cooling, nothing. Even on hot, dry days you need to adapt your routine and slow down.*

**Rehydrate:** In all hot weather, take frequent water breaks. Sweating can deplete your body's fluid reservoirs so it's vital to top them up with small quantities of cold water – before, during and after your workout (be sure to sip and not gulp). Keep drinking every 15 to 20 minutes to prevent dehydration: don't wait until you feel thirsty. Keep away from canned squashes: it is thought that glucose slows down absorption of fluid into the system. Replace lost potassium post-workout with orange or grapefruit juice or a banana.

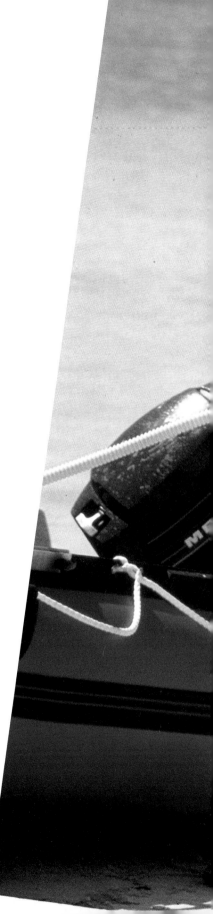

SUMMER ZEST

Cool exercise continued

**The vital cool-down:** *Remember to cool down gradually: reduce your pace and walk slowly for a while. Try and have a cool shower: merely mopping sweat with a towel won't lower your core temperature.*

**Take the heat off:** Don't be tempted to abandon your regular workout routine altogether. When the heat's off you'll be back in class or on the track feeling the strain! Follow these guidelines:

*Use common sense to gauge temperature and act accordingly. How soon do you feel hot and sticky when you get outdoors? If you're a confirmed jogger or play a sport, get out early in the morning, before the sun is up, or in the cool of the evening. This particularly applies to cities where heat bounces off buildings and hard surfaces causing even higher temperatures. If you're on holiday and aren't doing your usual class, take cool dips and* **swim** *yourself fit. Water soaks up several thousand times more heat than air of the same temperature, so makes swimming the ideal workout substitute on humid days.*

**Watchpoint:** *Overheated swimming pools create the same problems as sultry weather on dry land. You may sweat a bit when you are swimming, but the surrounding warm water will prevent evaporation.*

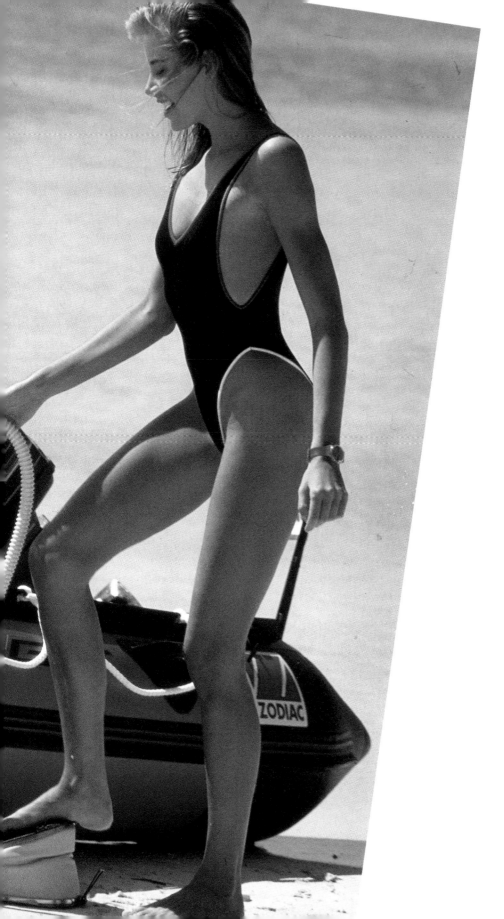

# SUMMER ZEST

Your body will adjust to summer temperature changes more easily if you've been taking regular, vigorous exercise year-round. But if summer is the time you zip into action, don't rush into your chosen activity. You'll need to give your body time to adapt to the new demands you're putting on it and to prevent muscle soreness and minor injuries.

**Watchpoint:** An air-conditioned aerobics studio will be cooler than an outdoor tennis court in the midday sun.

---

*Slow easy stretches are the ideal answer when you can't bear moving in the heat. The advantage of hot weather here: your muscles will already be warm and relaxed. But you'll still need to do warm-up exercises by walking on the spot and swinging your arms for a few minutes to stimulate your circulation and motor nerves for safer, more effective muscle function. Try the following three key positions for loosening your legs and hips. If you can, hold each stretch for at least 30 seconds to allow time for the tension in muscles to fully release; don't bounce or force the stretch. Take a deep breath and breathe deeply throughout the stretch. Concentrate on lengthening your body without forcing.*

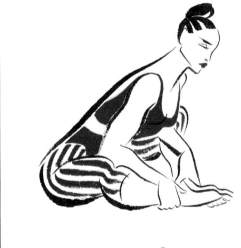

◀ ✳ GROIN, HIPS AND INNER THIGHS: Sit on towel, rug or mat. Start with soles of feet together, hands behind you for support. Try to lengthen your spine upwards from the crown of your head while you ease your knees gently outwards. Once you can hold your back up straight without support, hold your ankles and try to bend forwards gently from the hips to increase the stretch. After this stretch, shake your legs out well.

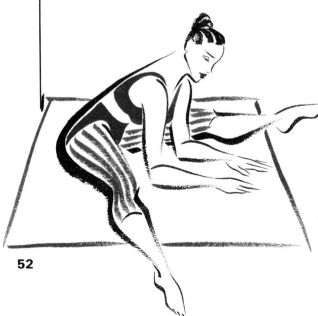

◀ ✳ THIGHS, HIPS AND GROIN: Sit with your legs wide apart. Lengthen your spine so that your back is straight, ribs and chest lifted and hip bones pushed forwards. Increase the stretch either by opening your legs wider or bending your

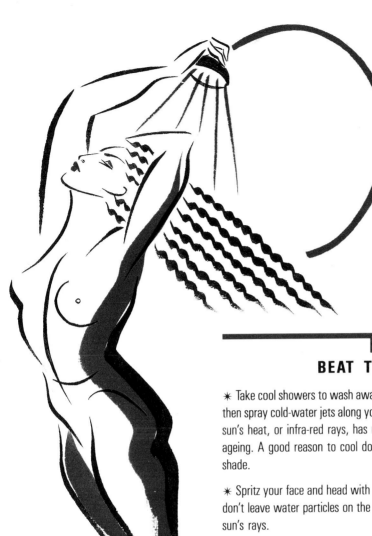

body forwards from the hips, while keeping your back flat. Shake your legs out and then bring them together so they are straight out in front of you for the third stretch.

∗ BACK OF THIGHS: Keep knees facing upwards and ankle bones together. Once you can sit up straight with backs of your knees on the ground, increase the stretch by bending forwards from hips and lengthening the body out along thighs.

## BEAT THE HEAT

∗ Take cool showers to wash away perspiration and reduce body heat, then spray cold-water jets along your spine to keep you cool longer. The sun's heat, or infra-red rays, has recently been linked with premature ageing. A good reason to cool down with a dip and make use of the shade.

∗ Spritz your face and head with refreshing cool water frequently. But don't leave water particles on the face, particularly – they magnify the sun's rays.

∗ If your body is well-hydrated, your urine will be light coloured and plentiful. If it's dark and scant, up your water intake. Plain, pure water is the liquid most quickly absorbed by the body.

∗ Soothe swollen legs. Beat summer heat with an ice pack by wrapping cubes in a cotton cloth and placing on legs/ankles . . . up to 5 minutes if you can bear it!

∗ Wear loose-fitting clothes – this will not only help you regulate your body temperature but will help you avoid skin pimples and sores under the breasts, caused by unevaporated perspiration. A fine dusting of talcum powder helps keep breasts dry.

∗ Keep a skin care sun kit with you during the day. Cotton wool discs, a cleanser and refreshing toner will combat skin breakouts caused by heat-stimulated sebum and help you keep your cool wherever you are – on the beach, heading out of the office for a meeting across town, or dashing out for the evening.

# *ZEST*

# Sunshine sports

Take a look at the body-shaping benefits of these outdoor sports and exercise activities. Summer is the perfect time to practise them. The smart way to boost your enjoyment of most sports and games is to take a few lessons before you jump straight in. That way you won't get disheartened (or feel foolish) but will be revved up with enthusiasm to improve your skills. The more competitive you are, the better the workout.

### Cycling

Fast becoming a cult, cycling is fantastic for shaping up the legs and buttocks. Some upper body exercise too for arms and shoulder muscles through steadying yourself in the saddle and gripping the handlebars. Excellent for improving aerobic fitness, and helpful for co-ordination.

### Horse-riding

*A tough workout for inner thigh and calf muscles, with the trunk muscles (stomach, waist, hips, back) constantly working to maintain balance. Develops balance and co-ordination, but does little for stamina and suppleness.*

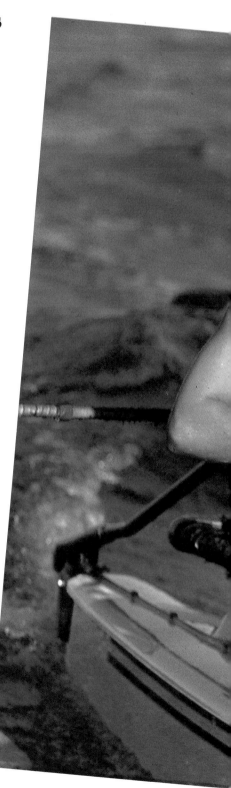

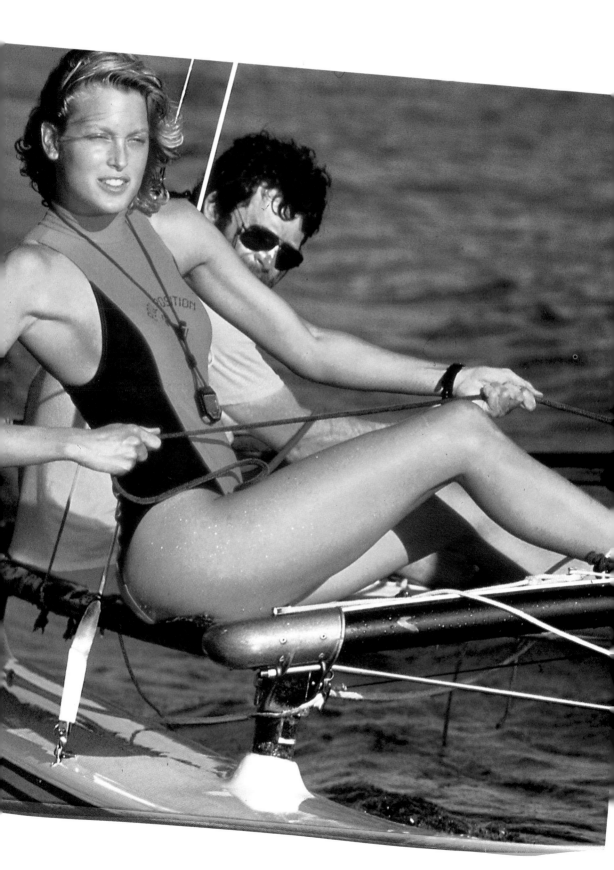

Sunshine sports continued

### Netball and basketball

The jumping and running strengthens legs (quads, calves, hamstrings), buttocks and upper body. Boosts aerobic fitness, co-ordination, and flexibility.

### Sailing

*Relaxing and easy-going unless you're sailing at a highly competitive level. Some arm and shoulder strengthening, although winches do the heavy work. If you go out on the trapeze, you'll develop your abdominals.*

### Swimming

Tones muscles in the upper body – arms, shoulders and trunk – and, to a lesser degree, the legs. Also improves aerobic fitness (excellent if your technique gets you through the water fast enough), flexibility and co-ordination. Tension can build up in the neck and shoulder muscles if you sustain breast-stroke, so practise freestyle (crawl) and backstroke as well.

### Tennis

*Some degree of proficiency is needed before you begin to see the physical benefits. Terrific for strengthening the muscles of the arms (especially the racquet arm, of course), shoulders, chest, waist and back. Good for co-ordination and improves flexibility to some extent. Keep moving to tone legs. Do extra stretching exercises to help your game and avoid pulling muscles. Aerobic benefits aren't huge – keep moving to increase your stamina.*

## TIPS FOR TINTING

Eyelash-tinting is a really worthwhile beauty investment, especially if you are blonde or red-headed. Have lashes (and eyebrows if you wish), tinted at least 3 to 4 days ahead of departure for a holiday destination. Although irritation is very rare, you want to be sure that there is no reaction before you go away, so don't leave it to the very last day. If you're a first-timer, you need to go to the salon 8 hours beforehand for a patch test. You can have this done first thing and then return later in the day for the actual tinting. Colours range from brown to darkest blue-black, the tinting takes 20 to 30 minutes and the effect lasts up to 12 weeks.

### Volleyball

You've got to be fit to play this sport! It makes strong demands on the lower body with constant jumping, diving, squatting and running. If you play as an attacker you will develop upper body strength. Excellent for co-ordination. Anaerobic at moderate levels of skill (depending on your aerobic fitness level). Do lots of stretching exercises, especially for the lower body.

### Waterskiing

*A real body-sculpting activity. You need strength in your legs (quads, calves), buttocks, arms, shoulders, back and stomach to stay up for any length of time. Does little for stamina or flexibility.*

### Windsurfing

Great fun if you're strong enough and can get to grips with the technique. Benefits: as for waterskiing.

# **L**earn to be graceful

Good posture, co-ordination and balance start with body awareness. We're often in such a hurry to get from A to B that we don't consider how we're using our bodies or think about enjoying the movement.

Unfortunately, the human body readily adapts to years of misuse, a slumped body line becoming comfortable and difficult to correct. Holding your body in a hunched position every day, with incorrect distribution of weight, will sap your energy and create potential health – especially back – problems. Tensions set in and your movements will lose fluidity and convey negative messages to those around you.

#### DEVELOP RHYTHM AND POISE

* *If you are tight and tense you can't be graceful. Do lots of stretching to become supple.*

* *If you want to slink across a room, choreographer Bruno Tonioli suggests watching models on the catwalk. At home, tape a line the length of a room and practise an elegant, sensual walk, slightly crossing one leg in front of the other. Not a style suited to striding out though!*

* *Posture should be supported from the stomach, Bruno advises. To help you know how it should feel, practise doing pliés. (See Dancers' Stretches on page 160).*

*If you are tight and tense you can't be graceful. Do lots of stretching to become supple.*

Learn to be graceful continued

✳ *Dance classes are a great way to awaken the grace in you. Try jazz before you sign up for ballet. Jazz classes combine dance routines with classical exercises. You'll increase your body confidence and rhythm before going on to more difficult balletic movements.*

✳ **Confidence builders:** *Clothes play an important role in determining how you move. You will hold yourself better in well-cut clothes, have body confidence instead of body-consiousness. Only buy clothes you feel fabulous in and choose comfortable shoes.*

# delicious healthy cocktails

**Raw juices** Freshly squeezed juices win out in the health and taste stakes. They lose their nutritional benefit quickly, however, so make only as much as you can drink immediately. If you have to, cover and refrigerate after squeezing to retain nutrients and flavour.

**Juice-extracting** *Use a traditional squeezer, a separator or an electric extractor. Separators can be used for soft fruits – although many are not suitable for citrus fruits – and are the only convenient way to make vegetable juice. If you don't want to invest in a juicer but have a blender, you can make fresh drinks from soft fruits. Simply chop up the fruits and add enough water (filtered or bottled is best, but not sparkling) to facilitate blending. Make a fruit 'slush' with crushed ice, or use natural yogurt for a satisfying, health-giving fruit shake.*

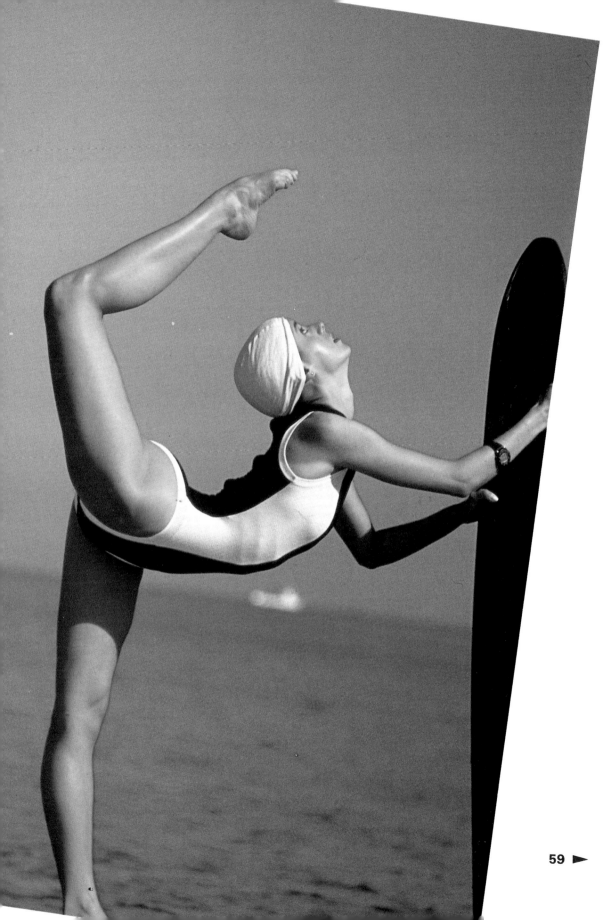

Delicious healthy cocktails continued

## SUMMER ZEST

**Which fruits to choose for delicious summer drinks?** Soft, almost over-ripe fruits are best; fruits such as papaya, banana and mango have high mineral contents and are good to use as natural sweeteners, instead of sugar or honey, with other more tart fruits. Taste-tempting blends to try: *mango and passionfruit; pineapple and orange; banana and pear. Berries such as raspberries, strawberries, cranberries, redcurrants and black currants, are very good with yogurt* – sprinkle chopped hazelnuts or almonds on top for added vitamin value.

**Citrus juices** *are heaped full of goodies needed for high-level health: vitamin C and small quantities of iron, which is effectively absorbed due to the presence of vitamin C; B1 which helps produce energy; pectin – a fibre that also reduces cholesterol.*

Perfect for sipping on the patio or balcony: fruit juice concentrates such as apricot, papaya or mango, mixed with chilled bubbly mineral water and garnished with a sprig of mint. You should always dilute concentrated juices.

**Vegetable juices** *are valuable sources of vitamins, minerals and enzymes. Carrot juice is also a very effective skin cleanser, digestive aid and infection fighter. A little lemon juice stops it going brown. Juices such as parsley, spinach and watercress are too trong or bitter to drink on their own and are best combined with another juice, such as carrot.*

### FAST TO FIX NON-ALCOHOLIC COCKTAILS:

### Reverend Davis
50 ml (2 fl oz) orange juice
juice of 1 lemon
dash of grenadine

Pour orange and lemon juice over ice and add grenadine.

### Fellini: a mock Bellini
50 ml (2 fl oz) peach nectar
50 ml (2 fl oz) non-alcoholic sparkling wine

Pour the nectar into a fluted glass and top up with the sparkling 'wine'.

### Peach and almond hammock
4 fresh peaches
50 g (2 oz) ground almonds
600 ml (1 pint) apple juice

Blend in a liquidizer and serve chilled.

*Melt-in-the-mouth strawberries, sharp, vibrant citrus, taste bud-challenging vegetables. Mix summer fruits and vegetables to make refreshing drinks that are rich in nutrients and doubly delicious.*

## Vegetable and fruit summer cocktail

3 parts carrot
1 part spinach
1 part watercress
1 part apple juice
6 ice cubes

Liquidize ingredients together and serve garnished with a slice of lime, orange and sprig of mint.

## Citrus cooler

1 cup of crushed ice
juice of ½ lime
25 ml (1 fl oz) plain low-fat yogurt
65 ml (2½ fl oz) orange juice
65 ml (2½ fl oz) pineapple juice
65 ml (2½ fl oz) grapefruit juice

Liquidize until smooth.

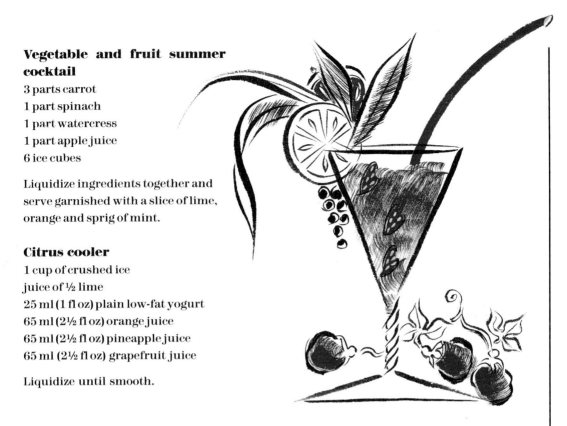

# nutritious fruit delights

Discover the super natural beauty boosters – fresh fruits that are rich sources of vitamins, minerals, fibre and carbohydrate. Indulge yourself in the tropical taste treats – try aromatic mangoes, guavas, and papayas. Best eaten raw, fruit is an important part of your diet. Mix your own exotic fruit combinations for breakfast and desserts, freshly pulped in delectable drinks and for the healthiest of snacks.

What to look for when choosing tropical fruit, and the lowdown on the nutrients in highest concentration, are listed on the following pages. (The fruits contain other vitamins and minerals too, but in smaller quantities.)

**Soft fruit** *This deteriorates very quickly, so is best eaten on the day of purchase or stored overnight in the refrigerator. Tropical fruit is best consumed within a few days of ripening. Most fruit can be frozen. Fruit should be undamaged and just ripe. If not, stew or purée the fruit first.*

**Dried fruit** Drying fruit concentrates its nutritional value. It is full of fibre, natural sugars, protein, vitamins A, B and C, calcium, iron, plus other minerals. Avoid sulphured fruits – they contain sulphur dioxide (E220) which can cause alimentary problems and destroys B vitamins. Wash before eating.

*ZEST*

Nutritious fruit delights continued

*VITAMIN A: Strengthens the skin and cell walls, protecting against infection, cancer and ageing.*

*VITAMIN B1: Needed to convert glucose into energy and in protein metabolism.*

*VITAMIN B2: Breaks down fats, carbohydrates and proteins for energy. Also required for cellular repair and growth.*

*VITAMIN B3: Active in energy production and for healthy skin.*

*VITAMIN B6: Involved in the metabolism of amino acids and proteins. Alleviates pre-menstrual problems. (Women are often deficient in it.)*

*VITAMIN B12: Essential for the production of red blood cells and healthy nerves.*

*FOLIC ACID: Also a B vitamin. Needed to make RNA and DNA. Important in early pregnancy.*

*Discover the super natural beauty boosters – fresh fruits that are rich sources of vitamins, minerals, fibre and carbohydrate.*

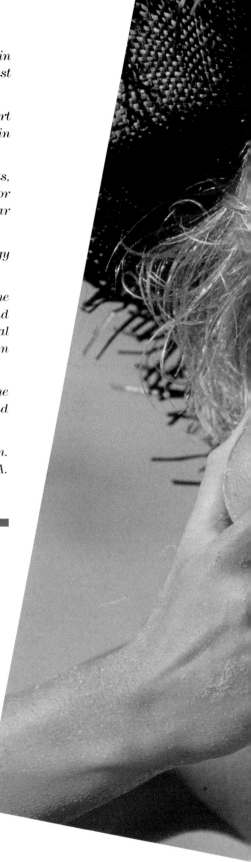

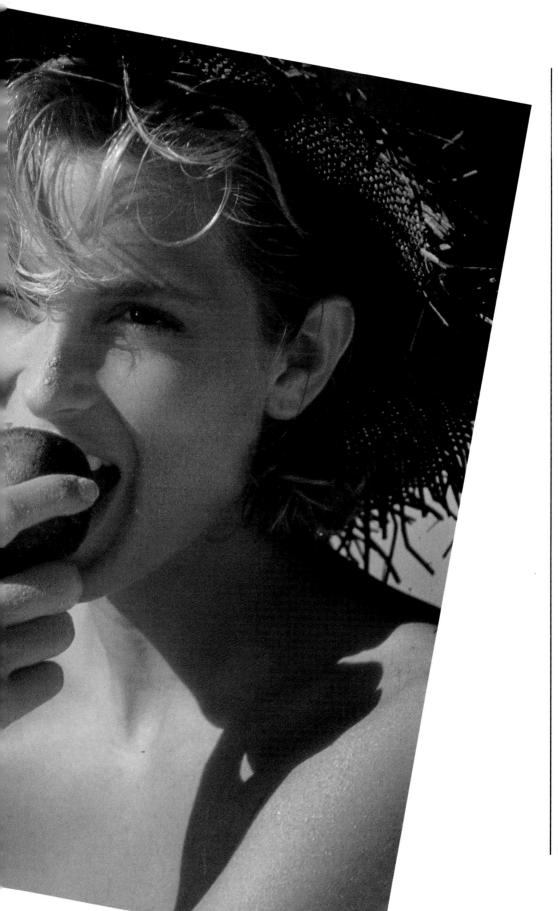

VITAMIN C: Essential for the formation of antibodies and for healing. Helps form collagen. Has a vital role as an anti-oxidant and is also needed for absorbing iron and producing haemoglobin.

VITAMIN E: Protects vitamins A, C and D and unsaturated fatty acids in the body from oxidation, thereby protecting against cell damage. Assists in healing and can provide protection against circulatory problems.

MAGNESIUM, CALCIUM AND PHOSPHORUS: Important for the skeletal and nervous system.

SODIUM AND POTASSIUM: Regulate body fluids.

ZINC: Important for growth and repair of tissues and the body's defence system. Deficiency can result in fatigue.

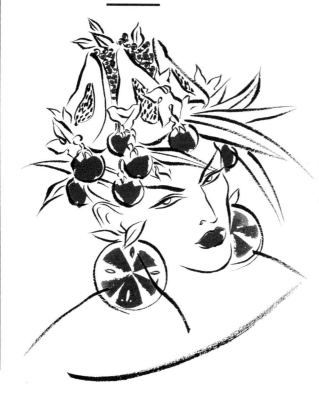

## APRICOT

**P**acked with vitamin A, apricots are frequently unripe when you buy them, so simply leave them on a window ledge for a few days. Ripe apricots should be refrigerated. You can remove the skin by first washing, then pouring boiling water over the fruit and leaving for 10 minutes. Brushing with lemon juice will stop them from going brown. Choose firm, golden fruit.

Dried apricots have the highest protein level of all dried fruit and are an excellent source of vitamin A and potassium, with some vitamin B2. They can be eaten as they are or soaked for a few hours until they expand.

## BANANA

*A good source of magnesium and potassium. Brush with a little lemon juice to prevent browning when adding to fruit salads. Great as a snack because they're very filling. Choose firm yellow fruit with no black marks.*

Dried bananas come whole, sliced lengthwise or as banana pieces. Dried whole and sliced bananas are very sweet but better for you than banana chips which are pieces of unripe banana deep-fried in sugar and oil.

## GUAVA

Usually round or pear-shaped with yellow skins. Strongly aromatic fruits with vivid red or pink flesh filled with pips (like a tomato). Peel off the skin and eat flesh and pips. Use lemon juice to prevent discoloration. A good source of vitamin C.

## KIWIFRUIT

*Rich in vitamin C, kiwifruit are a colourful garnish for fruit salads. Peel off the skin, slice and eat raw. The fruits should yield to slight pressure when touched.*

## KUMQUAT

A tiny citrus fruit. You eat the whole fruit, including the skin which is usually sweeter than the flesh. Kumquats contain vitamin A. Look for small, bright orange fruit.

## MANGOE

*There are many varieties of mango with different shapes and colours. A good source of vitamin A. Cut lengthwise and remove the stone. Aromatic, a real summer treat.*

## MELON

There are many different types of melon. Cantaloupes are a good source of vitamin A, with 2000 mcg per 100 g (4 oz); they also contain some folic acid. Round, with ribbed, dark green skins and orange flesh. Look for firm fruit and use fingertip pressure around the base to test for ripeness. Smell the melon as it may have a light scent when it's ready for eating. For watermelons, look for a dull (not shiny) skin.

## PAPAYA/PAW PAW

*With their bright pink flesh and wonderful aromatic sweetness, papayas make a wonderful mid-summer breakfast alternative to grapefruit. They are well-stocked with vitamin A and contain some zinc. Oval-shaped and narrower at one end, you should look for papayas with no soft spots or blemishes which give evenly under gentle pressure.*

## PASSION FRUIT/ GRANADILLA

Eat the tangy, heavily scented seeds of passion fruit and you're providing your body with fibre, protein, and some vitamin B2. They also contain sodium (salt) – useful on dehydrating hot sultry days. Look for firm, heavy fruit with slightly wrinkled skins. Cut the hard shell with a sharp knife. If you prefer to skip the pips, pass through a sieve.

## PERSIMMON/SHARON FRUIT

*To look at, the sharon fruit resembles a large orange-coloured tomato. Pull away the stalk, cut in half and inside you'll find very sweet orange flesh. When ripe, they're very soft to touch. Contain vitamin A, C, iron and calcium.*

SUMMER *ZEST*

## PINEAPPLE

Containing an enzyme called bromelin, believed to be able to break down fats, pineapples contain some vitamin A and C, potassium, calcium and magnesium. The fruit should yield gently to fingertip pressure and have a pleasant scent when ripe. You can also test if they are ready to eat by pulling a leaf out of the crown – if it comes away easily it should be ripe. Remove the black marks with the skin because they can irritate the skin and mouth. Cut the core out if it is very tough and fibrous.

## POMEGRANATE

*Delicious and refreshing, pomegranates contain potassium magnesium and calcium. Look for even-coloured, heavy fruit. Cut a slice off at the stem end and section. Bend back the skin and enjoy the juicy red seeds.*

# hot hints for no-sweat make-up

✳ Hot weather activates oil and perspiration glands, often resulting in whiteheads and blackheads. At the same time sun, salt and chlorine can dry your skin, making it rough and flaky. For a healthy and clear complexion, cleanse your face frequently with a non-drying product. Exfoliate daily with a washcloth or weekly with a mild facial scrub, unless your skin has broken out (you might spread the infection). Deep-clean pores with a mask once a week or more often when needed.

✳ Switch to a lighter moisturizer and check it has UV screens. Look out for oil-free formulations.

✳ Some cosmetic houses make 'blotting' lotions which combat the shiny centre panel. Choose a foundation with a higher water content and less oil for hot weather wear. Oil melts in heat to become sticky and shiny.

✳ Spritz your face with a mist of water (kept in the refrigerator) to give your foundation a dewy finish or for a fast refresher during the day.

✳ Eye make-up creases quickly in humid atmospheres. Make sure lids are dry before applying shadow by dusting with a little translucent powder. Look out for waterproof eyeshadows and blushers.

*For a healthy and clear complexion, cleanse your face frequently with a non-drying product.*

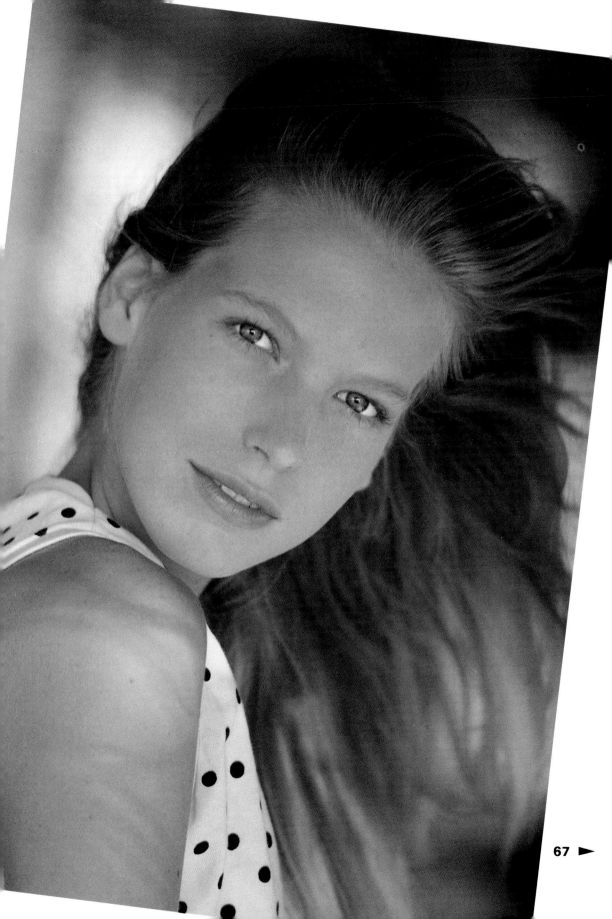

SUMMER ZEST

## FEATHERWEIGHT MOUSSE MAKE-UP

The new generation of mousses has taken to make-up, making fresh and translucent-looking foundations, blushers and concealers. They're the perfect featherweight, airy option for summer, and – if you know the knack – easy to apply.

✳ Apply mousse make-up on to moisturized skin. Otherwise its high powder content can look patchy, or settle into fine lines.

✳ Apply mousse concealer before foundation.

✳ Mousse foundations usually need no extra powder dusted on top to set them, unless you want a very matte finish or have an oily centre panel, when you may wish to apply a little to the T-zone – the forehead, nose and chin.

✳ To get a glowing, even hint of colour with mousse blusher, mix it with a tiny amount of moisturizer before applying, then smooth on a little at a time.

# hotshot hair removers

**Q.** *My skin often becomes irritated after my legs have been waxed. Why is this? Is there any way to prevent it?*

**A.** The skin becomes irritated after waxing because of stress caused to the hair follicles when the hairs are pulled out, which makes the skin prone to small breakouts.

Waxing is nevertheless a good hair-removal method for legs and bikini area – it needs to be repeated less often than shaving or using depilatory creams, and the hair often grows back more slowly and finer in texture.

✳ Proper techniques can minimize irritation both during and after a wax treatment. The wax shouldn't be too hot and the skin should be stretched as taut as possible as the wax is removed. Waxing should never be done over skin that is already irritated, broken or abrased. Salon waxing is your best option for delicate skin on the face, particularly the upper lip, and for hard-to-reach areas like the under

*Waxing should never be done over skin that is already irritated, broken or abrased.*

arms and bikini line, where the hair may also grow in several directions. Repeatedly removing the hairs at the wrong angle can distort the follicles, making future removal more difficult. If you break the hair off at the surface instead of removing it at the roots, the effect will not last long.

* The most popular type of waxing is the cool wax method, where the wax is removed with a gauze strip. With hot wax, which some people report is less painful, the wax is stripped off when it has cooled and solidified on the skin, then filtered and re-used on the next client. In view of today's heightened awareness of hygiene, it is wise to check that the salon is using the cool wax system.

* To avoid further irritation of the hair follicles you need to be a little careful for 24 hours after waxing. Skip sun exposure and strenuous activity, don't use heavy or greasy moisturizers, under-arm (if you've been waxed there) deodorants, or products containing alcohol or fragrance. Take cool, not hot, showers, and wait a day before going swimming in salt or chlorinated water, using a whirlpool or having a massage.

* Finally, try smoothing on a non-irritant lotion, with a soothing ingredient such as allantoin – ask the salon to recommend one.

Q. *I'm considering having electrolysis on the dark hairs above my lip. What does electrolysis actually consist of? How painful will it be and how long will the effects of electrolysis last?*

A. First, ensure that electrolysis is done only by a specialist. Look around for someone who has plenty of experience, and ensure that the salon uses disposable needles. Never use kits designed for at-home electrolysis – you could cause irreparable scarring and skin damage.

* Sensitivity to pain varies greatly: some people are only able to have a few hairs removed at each session; others feel little pain. In general, it is quite painful on the face. On average, 15 hairs are removed at each visit. After an initial consultation, the sessions usually take about 15 minutes.

* Never pluck hairs above the lip; if you do this, or have waxed them, this can make electrolysis more difficult as the hair follicles may be distorted. It is advisable to have electrolysis done as soon as dark hair appears. Don't bleach the hair immediately before treatment – it makes the skin extra-sensitive and the hair difficult to see. An electrolysist will not remove hairs from a mole or from areas of pigmented skin.

* There will be some reddening and puffiness after treatment, so don't schedule your appointment before a business meeting or evening out. If your skin is oily, the heat can stimulate sebum and small pimples may form. Your electrolysist may suggest an antiseptic lotion to help heal them.

* Treatments will be spread out over a number of months or years as hair follicles have dormant periods and you need to catch each

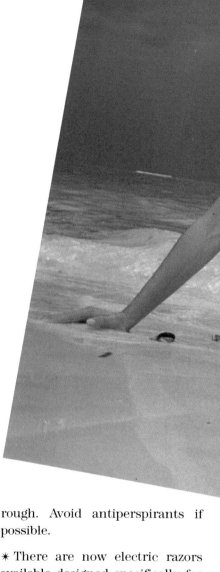

follicle in an active cycle. This method of hair removal is permanent, though hormonal changes at a future date may result in new hair growth.

✳ Areas other than the lip that are often treated with electrolysis include brows and other facial hair and the bikini line (the latter is particularly expensive).

**Q.** *Is there a trick to rash-free shaving?*

**A.** Shaving sloughs off the skin's outer layer, leaving it less protected against potential irritants such as elasticated swimsuit edges which can rub the bikini line; soreness can be triggered by perspiration, alcohol and para-amino benzoic acid (PABA) in sunscreens, salt water, chlorine and sand.

✳ *The rash-free solution*: Shave the afternoon before you hit the beach/poolside to give skin time to recover, but not for shadow to appear.

✳ Don't shave just before you rush off to a party/meeting. If you're hurrying, chances are you'll get a nasty nick which could scar.

✳ When shaving under the arms, you may find they sting afterwards due to razor burn – a series of small cuts and abrasions on the skin. *Preventive measure*: Use a shaving cream that's rich in emollients to ensure your razor glides over the skin, use a sharp blade and preferably a gentle razor with a comb guard. A man's razor or a cheap disposable razor are likely to be too rough. Avoid antiperspirants if possible.

✳ There are now electric razors available designed specifically for the delicate bikini line.

✳ When shaving your legs, shaving from the knee down does not give as close a shave as shaving from the ankle up, against the

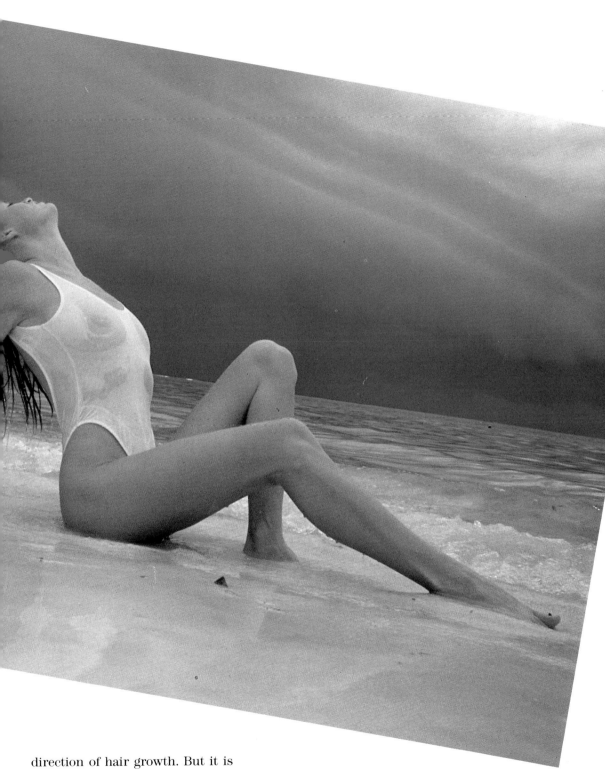

direction of hair growth. But it is
less likely to cause irritation. Try
using a cream bleach to lighten
hairs on your thighs and avoid the
time and hassle of extra shaving.

**Q.** *How should I remove the fine hairs around my nipples?*

**A.** Plucking, shaving and waxing the hairs around nipples can cause irritation and infection and therefore shouldn't be done. Instead, trim them with scissors. Electrolysis is the once-and-for-all solution (*except* for pigmented areas) but can be uncomfortable.

* If you have dark hairs between your breasts, bleach them with a gentle product.

**Q.** *What other at-home options are there for removing the hair from my legs, apart from shaving?*

**A.** Waxing is usually done more efficiently by a beauty salon. The results last for several weeks; odd hairs that were not long enough or were at the beginning of the growth cycle will become more visible before the rest of the hair grows back and can be removed with depilatory creams or by shaving.

* Depilatory creams dissolve the hair just below the skin surface and the results last longer than shaving. Always do a patch test 24 hours before using a new product.

* There is a new electrical beauty product worth considering. Designed for removing hairs on the legs (it should not be used under the arms or on the bikini line), the hand-held unit has a spinning wire spiral that plucks hairs from the legs as you sweep it over the surface. Results are long-lasting and some testers found it less painful, and more convenient, than waxing. It is available from selected department stores and chemists.

# Summer survival

### SAND IN YOUR EYE

**S**unglasses provide some protection against wind-swept sandy beaches. Nevertheless, sand can easily get in your eye. *Treatment*: Wash the eye straight away. Dunk your head in the water and allow the grit to float away. If it doesn't, don't rub your eye – you could scratch the eye's surface and increase the damage. Lift your head, blink rapidly and pull your upper eyelid gently down, let it go and dunk your head again. Try several times and if you can't remove the sand, head for the doctor's office or emergency ward immediately – it could be lodged on your cornea, and if so will need expert help. If it is trapped under your lid or on the white of the eye, a doctor will lift it away with a sterile swab.

*Prevent a painful rash or sting spoiling your fun this summer.*

## SUMMER PESTS

*Sand flies* Tiny pests, often found along the beach edge. They breed in holes in trees and get active early morning and night.

*Mosquitoes* breed in fresh water pools, attack all day and liven up in the evening.

*Sand fleas* Most active at dawn and dusk. Keep all at bay with a repellant. Avoid contact with eyes and lips, swimsuits or clothing. Re-apply every 2 hours, as the sun hots up the rate of evaporation.

Avoid scents – apart from causing sun sensitivity problems, they are believed to attract pests, so watch out at sunset beach barbecues. Check too that your sunscreen is not scented.

*Treatment:* If you are bitten, there are many over-the-counter pain and itch relievers. Some ingredients can cause sensitivity and if you break out in an allergic-type, itchy rash, avoid them in future. Look for antiseptic ingredients to kill off any bacteria that might breed in the broken skin and try not to scratch. You could push any germs present into the skin and delay the healing process.

### 'SAND' RASH

*An itchy rash caused by hookworm larvae in tropical zones. It may appear several hours or even weeks after the hookworm has burrowed under the skin. The itching can be so intense you'll likely head straight to the doctor who will prescribe a quick relief remedy. The larvae live in the intestines of dogs and transfer to the sand through excrement. Stick to beaches which are cleaned frequently if you can, wear shoes for walking, and use a rubber mat or folding chair for*

*Sunglasses provide some protection against wind-swept sandy beaches. Nevertheless, sand can easily get in your eye.*

*sunning – these bugs can burrow through a damp towel!*

### SEA URCHIN SPINES

Found on rocky, not sandy, sea beds, the spines can be tricky to remove. *Treatment*: Using tweezers, pull the spines out gently and slowly in the direction the spine went in to avoid breaking it. A mild acid, like vinegar, can help dissolve pieces of the spine left behind but if you suspect any are left in the skin, call a doctor. Sea urchins produce toxins that can cause painful swelling and the broken skin may become infected.

Once the spines are out, reduce any swelling and pain by holding ice cubes to the area for 10 minutes every few hours. Hydrocortisone cream eases inflammation and an antibacterial product will protect against infection.

### STINGS

∗ *Bicarbonate of soda (baking powder) dissolved in a little water eases bee stings. Use a weak acid solution – lemon juice or vinegar in water – for wasp stings.*

73 ▶

## SUMMER ZEST

* *Jellyfish with tentacles always sting, those without may or may not. Treatment: Deactivate any stingers, or nematocysts, that remain on the skin. Don't take a shower – tap water triggers the stingers to produce toxins. Lather up with sea-water and soap. Calamine lotion soothes the burning sensation and hydrocortisone cream helps relieve swelling and inflammation. The area will be swollen and sore for several days, depending on the severity of the sting and the type of jellyfish.*

*It is rare, but you could be allergic to jellyfish stings if you have symptoms of overall swelling, severe stomach cramps, faintness and difficulty in breathing. This kind of reaction can be fatal, so call an ambulanace and get to a hospital fast.*

*Take care to avoid dead jellyfish or tentacles on the beach. They can still sting.*

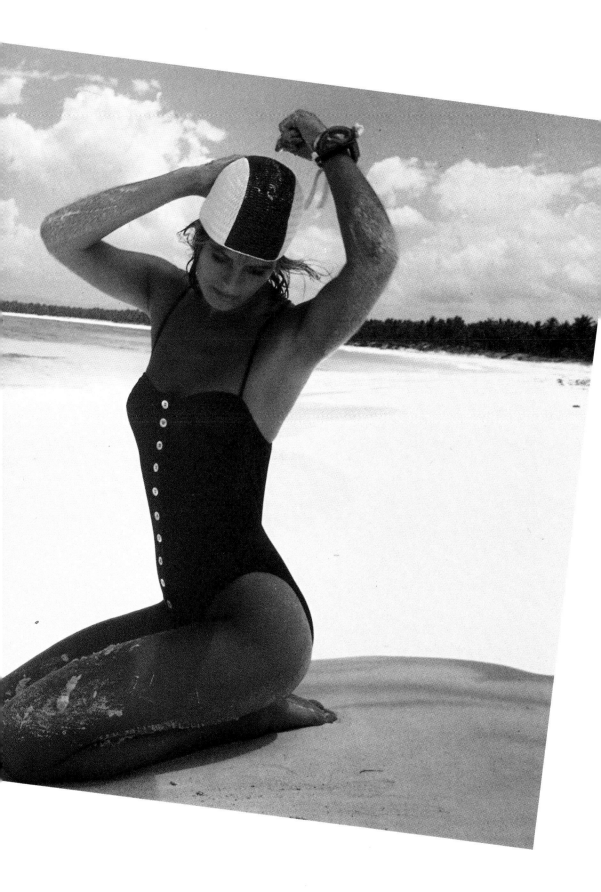

# **W**arm weather styles

**K**eep your hair looking sharp while you stay cucumber-cool with these fix-in-a-flash ideas for mid-length and long hair.

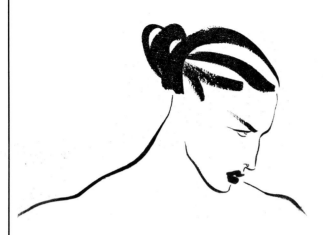

1. Simple chignon: a soft version of the slick classic that's chic for summer city days. Ideal for mid-length hair that's wavy or layered. Apply mousse to give hair added control. Gather your hair into a ponytail and secure with a covered elastic. Twist and grip with hair pins. Spray with hairspray if you need to.

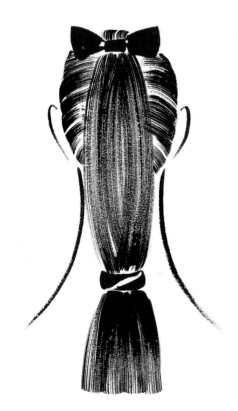

2. Slide style: Great for long hair. Using 2 differently coloured slides of the same design: one to secure hair in a half ponytail, another to grip hair mid-way between nape and end of hair.

*Fun, new ponytail style: first tie one ribbon into a bow. Then add a second in another colour.*

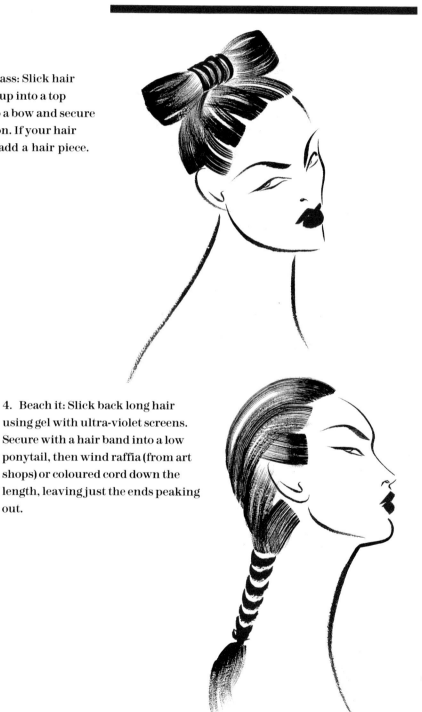

3. Summer night sass: Slick hair with gel and brush up into a top ponytail. Twist into a bow and secure with pins and ribbon. If your hair isn't long enough, add a hair piece.

4. Beach it: Slick back long hair using gel with ultra-violet screens. Secure with a hair band into a low ponytail, then wind raffia (from art shops) or coloured cord down the length, leaving just the ends peaking out.

# **S**leek feet

**The perfect pedicure:** Summer feet are on show. Treat your feet to a soothing, smoothing pedicure and keep up the good work about once a week.

*1.* *Remove old polish.*
*2.* *Soak feet for 15 minutes in soapy water (or invest in a soothing foot bath and check the timing on the package) or in warm water with a few drops of almond oil.*
*3.* *Dry thoroughly. Unless cuticles are growing up over the nail, it's better to leave them as they are. If they need help, apply cuticle remover and push them back very gently with a stick wrapped with cotton wool.*
*4.* *While nails are still soft, clip straight across just at the end of the toes. Use a metal clipper that won't leave sharp edges, and lightly file if necessary. Leave the sides unfiled to avoid painful ingrowing toenails.*

*Summer feet are on show. Keep them polished and neat with an at-home pedicure about once a week.*

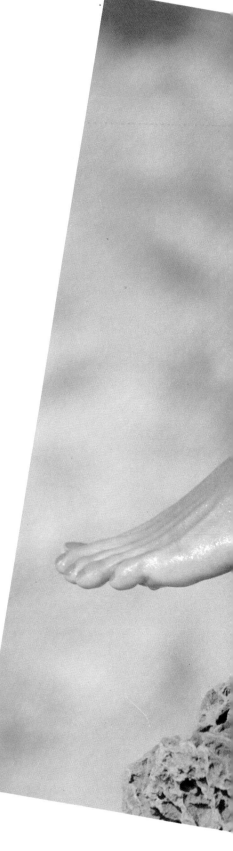

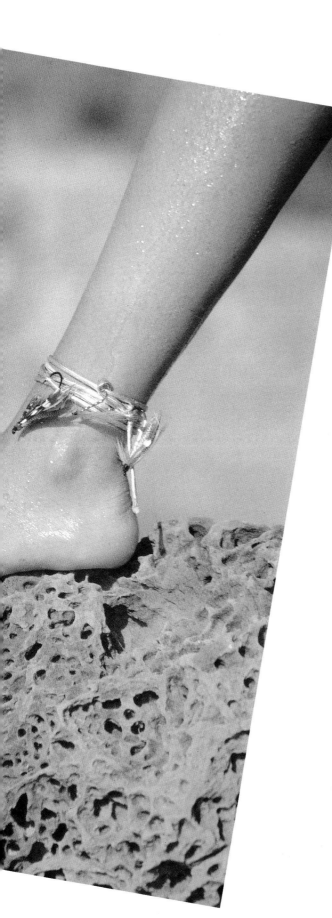

**5.** *Don't try to cut hard skin on soles of feet – you could inflict permanent damage. Carefully smooth any calluses with a foot file or pumice stone, or go to a chiropodist.*

**6.** *Lightly massage feet with a moisturizing hand, body or foot cream.*

**7.** *Apply polish: a base coat, followed by 2 coats of nail colour, finishing with a top coat.*

If your feet have been neglected for some time, invest in a professional pedicure to remove calluses and hard skin. You can buy at-home debumpers and skin smoothers – some are tougher on skin than others. Work on the safe side, smoothing the surface with a few strokes in one direction after soaking the feet. As soon as a corn or callus feels smoother, stop. Keep instruments scrupulously clean.

Bacteria or viruses can enter through dry, cracked skin so apply moisturizer after bathing. For a deep-moisturizing treatment, massage cream into your feet, cover them with plastic bags and warm towels for 5–10 minutes and relax.

# lunch quickies

How to be sure you don't miss lunch when deadlines keep you tied to the desk, or the weather's too bad to brave heading outside for a sandwich: Brown-bag your lunch to the office. Ten minutes in the morning (or before you go to bed) can save queuing for half an hour at lunchtime when you could be reading a book, taking a walk in the park, or chatting to a friend instead.

Best health bets for mid-day: balance carbohydrates (bread, potatoes and fruit) with low-fat protein (turkey, chicken, tuna, prawns, a hard-boiled egg, a wedge of low-fat cheese, scoop of low-fat yogurt or milk drink). Try pitta bread as a change from brown bread sandwiches. Make your own taramasalata – the home-produced version will be colouring-free. Fix a raw vegetable and fruit salad: eating two smaller, side salads for lunch and dinner will save you ploughing through one larger one in the evening. Pack salad dressing separately, or simply squeeze on a slice of lemon.

## NAIL IT! COLOUR CUES AND MANICURE TIPS

∗ How to choose polish colour when they all look inviting? Hold the bottle against the back of your hand.

∗ Pale colours do for fingers and hands what toning your shoes to your stockings does for your legs – slims, lengthens, flatters.

∗ Take top coat under nail tip to help prevent colour chipping and to strengthen the tip.

∗ When using a dark colour, always paint the strokes lengthwise beginning with centre stroke, then one along each side.

∗ *French manicure:* Paint the tip with white enamel, matte or pearlized. Better than nail pencil – keeps nails looking fresh and clean and gives them extra strength at tips where they need it. Repeat when dry with another tip coat.

∗ Buffing stimulates circulation. Use gentle strokes in the same direction.

∗ Nail polishes and hardeners which contain formaldehyde can cause sensitivity reactions on skin from touching your face, especially around the eyes. Look for formaldehyde-free formulations.

∗ False tips and nail-building techniques must be done by professionals. If the nails aren't completely dry or if an airlock is made when the resins are applied, fungal growths can occur. Salons will advise you about up-keep of nail extensions. If you can't commit yourself to returning for regular 'fill-ins', the nails can catch and break at the nail bed. Never remove tips yourself – you may damage the nail.

# **e**ye soothers

### CONJUNCTIVITIS

**H**ot, dry weather increases the chances of conjunctivitis (inflammation of the eyelid lining). Often due to viral or bacterial infection, sometimes caused by chlorine in swimming pools or infected dust in the eyes; allergic conjunctivitis often recovers spontaneously. Seek treatment as viral conjunctivitis can recur.

Don't use eye-washes or drops. Although they may help the symptoms, they could mask the cause and thus hinder recovery.

### *PUFFINESS*

*If you often wake up with puffy eyes, poor lymphatic drainage may be the cause. Tap on an eye gel formulated to soothe puffiness using the fourth (ring) finger – this has the lightest touch. Look for eye gel containing ingredients such as elderflower, marigold, camomile and witchhazel. Short-lived puffiness around the eyes is often caused by premenstrual water retention. Try sleeping with an extra pillow prior to your period so that your head is raised. Wake up early to give any puffiness time to go down and apply cool compresses such as ice cubes wrapped in cloth, cucumber or refrigerated potato slices, or use an eye mask which can be kept in the fridge. Seek medical attention for persistent puffiness that does not improve and is accompanied by pain, tenderness or redness, or that occurs in just one eye.*

*Follow these easy suggestions and keep your eyes sparkling.*

### VDU SIDE-EFFECTS

**V**DU users have been shown to suffer twice the normal incidence of eye discomfort. If you find working at a VDU is causing eyestrain, consult your optician. Special tinted glass lenses are available; however, if the VDU has a filter fitted this could cause extra problems.

### *SUNGLASSES*

*Short-sighted people are more affected by the sun's rays than normal-sighted people, because their pupils are less able to contract and*

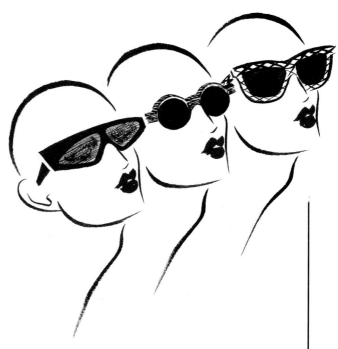

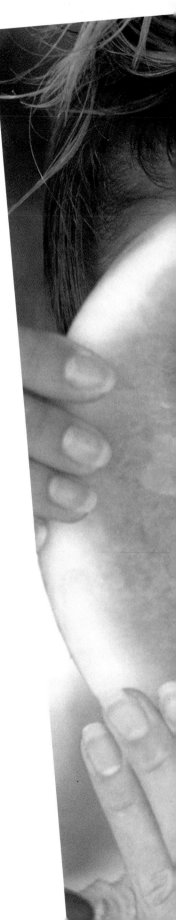

**SUMMER ZEST**

Eye soothers continued

protect the retina. Good sunglasses
will be particularly important in
such cases. On the whole, the more
expensive the glasses the better the
lenses. Poor quality lenses are
actually worse than nothing at all:
the pupils expand to let in more
light, reducing the barrier to
potentially damaging UV rays. If
you're spending a lot of time on the
water, choose semi-mirrored or
mirrored glasses to cut down
reflection.

Your best bet if you're clocking
up miles in the car or riding a
motorcycle are specialized driving
lenses. While virtually all lenses
are shatterproof now, some are
balanced to screen rays reflected
off road surfaces. Be wary when
you're wearing sunglasses or
tinted lenses for driving. Head into
a tunnel and you could be in
danger because the eyes take up to
a minute to adjust to the change in
light. Never wear tinted lenses for
driving at night.

**Which lens shade to choose?**
On a cloudy day there is a pre-
dominance of blue light which
makes everything appear grey
and objects in the distance
obscure. An amber tint cuts down
the level of blue light and increases
contrast. Choose dark green or
brown lenses for very bright sunlight.

**Sports fans:** Some sunglasses are
specially toughened to be impact-
resistant. Also available now: contact lenses with UV filters –
designed with action in mind.

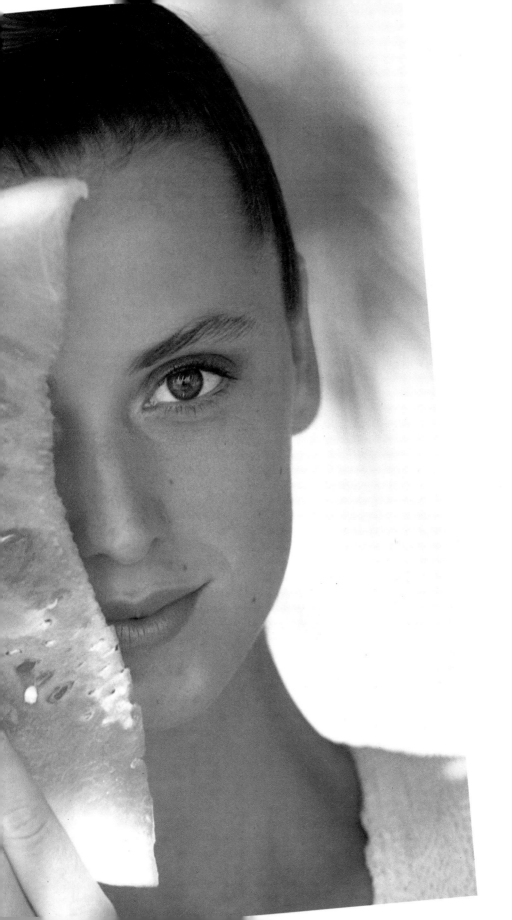

# travel tips

### COMBAT DEHYDRATION

✳ Pressurized cabin air is dry and dehydrating. Save your skin by removing your make-up, spritzing with water and applying an emollient cream. Take a mini plant spray with you or a mineral water spray (as long as it's in hand luggage). If you prefer not to take off your make-up, use a heavier than usual moisturizer, such as a night cream, underneath.

✳ Contact lens wearers will either need to take their lenses out during the flight or use special drops.

✳ Avoid alcohol, and coffee and tea which are diuretics. Don't drink alcohol the night before or in-flight but have lots of water and some fruit juice instead. Because of the exhausting effects of dehydra-

tion from alcohol, hangovers in the air can be 3 times worse than on the ground.

---

### OTHER IN-FLIGHT HAZARDS

✳ *Sitting for long periods combined with the speeded-up gravitational pull of the aeroplane, affects circulation and can produce fluid retention in tissues. Wear loose-fitting shoes and don't take them off during the flight (your feet will swell during a long-haul flight). Rest with your feet raised before you go to sleep, if possible. Use a soothing eye gel with ingredients that reduce puffiness – puffy eyes will make you look even more tired when you disembark.*

---

### FIGHTING JET-LAG

✳ You're headed for a four-hour time difference? Then it's likely you'll be affected by jet-lag. You may feel revved up when you need to sleep, feel drugged when you wake up. You may crave food at odd times or feel too sick to eat. Going East will double the effect of travelling West. If you're headed North or South, however, you won't hit the jet-lag problems.

Try these tips:

✳ Eating when your body thinks it's 3 a.m. is a bad move. Eat less than usual in the air – it's an opportunity to give your digestive system a break, too. Make a note saying 'Don't wake for meals'. Where mealtimes are in synch with regular eating patterns order

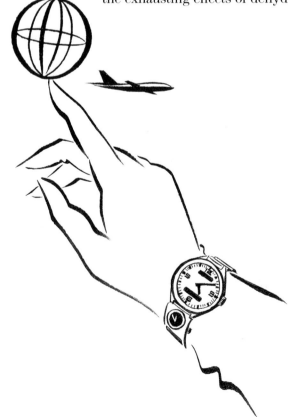

healthy food such as vegetarian or low-sodium meals if you're on a scheduled flight.

✳ If you've got to go into immediate action at your destination, try the advice of an American scientist: eat a high-protein meal (fish, poultry, eggs, yogurt, cheese, pulses and nuts) at the normal breakfast-time for your new base and a high-protein lunch. Eat a high-carbohydrate dinner (pasta, potatoes) several hours before you retire. Don't cat-nap during the day but retire fairly early.

✳ If you're arriving in the daytime, schedule an outdoor activity when you touch down. Bright light appears to minimize jet-lag. Many frequent travellers recommend physical activity – they say it increases their energy reserves. If you arrive in the evening, you could go for a walk or out dancing.

✳ Research is being done into the reduced levels of natural electro-magnetic waves that arise during jet travel and the effects on our circadian rhythm. Products are now being introduced which generate waves, reproducing the patterns you would find at ground level.

## TRAVEL KIT CHECKLIST

*In your hand luggage*:

Moisturizer
Make-up remover
Toner
Perfume atomizer
Toothpaste and travel toothbrush
Tissues
Mirror
Hairbrush/comb
Sunglasses and case
Small water spray
Eye mask (for long journeys)
Ear plugs
Fruit
Mineral water
Travel sickness remedies
Blusher
Eye pencils and mascara
Lipstick (and brush)

*In your suitcase or check-in bag*:

Sun protection for face, body, eyes and lips
After-sun moisturizer/soother
Shower gel
Shampoo and conditioner
Deep-conditioning hair treatment
Mousse/gel
Gel screen for hair

Hat/scarf
Travel hairdryer and multi-point adaptor
File, nail buffer and paste
Polish and remover
Cotton wool
Cotton buds
Face mask
Tweezers
Wide-toothed comb
Concealer in a darker colour than usual (for your tan)
Tinted moisturizer or foundation
Translucent loose powder
Waterproof mascara, eyeshadows and blusher
Waterproof make-up remover

*Small medical kit*:

Plasters
Scissors
Antiseptic lotion/ointment
Insect repellant
Calamine lotion
Upset stomach tablets
Antihistamine cream
Prescription medicines
Aspirin
Medical insurance and vaccination details

# Sun savvy

Light includes ultraviolet wavelengths of UVA, UVB and UVC. UVC rays are screened by the earth's atmosphere. UVB rays tan us and are the burning culprits. UVA's reach deeper into the skin and are also linked to ageing and cancer. In high doses, for instance in sun beds, UVA can tan and burn the skin.

Choose a product that has both UVA and UVB sunscreens. One popular screen, PABA or para-amino benzoic acid, can cause an allergic reaction – rough, red and itchy skin. The inflamed skin can be soothed with a hydrocortisone cream (containing no higher than 1% hydrocortisone).

*We tend, mistakenly, to gauge the burning power of the sun by the heat (infra-red rays) we feel. Be wary of cloudy days and when a breeze lowers the temperature – you can burn.*

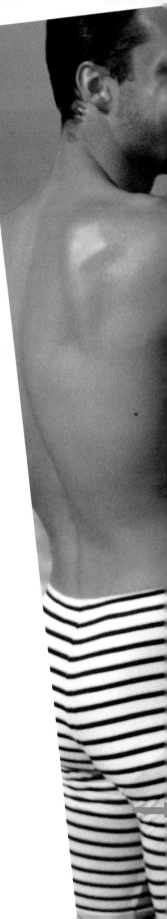

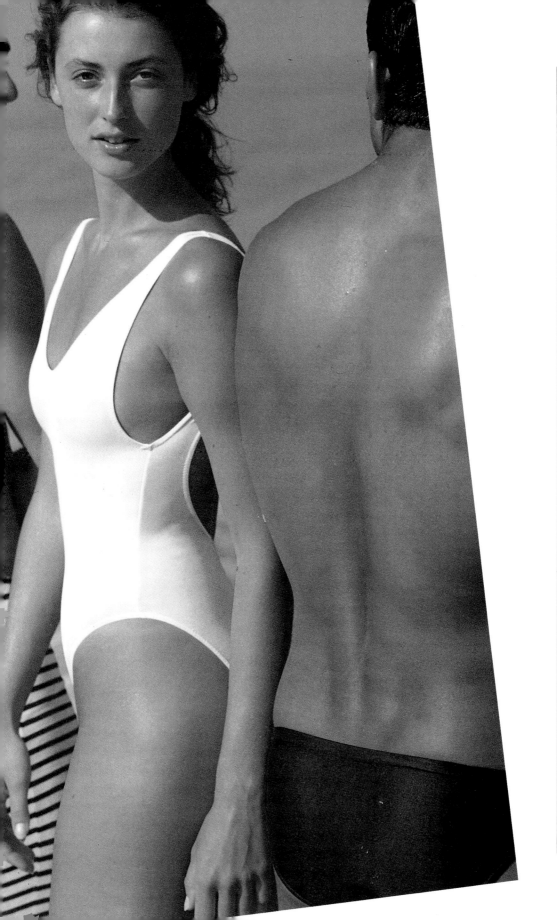

***How Sun Protection Factors (SPFs) work:*** *Protective products are labelled with either an SPF or factor number. An SPF 4 will let you stay out for 4 times as long compared to skin-singe time if you had not applied sun protection. However, at present, there is no international agreement governing the method of estimating an SPF, and products which carry a factor number, labelled, say, Factor 8, have undergone a different testing procedure.*

*A dermatologist's advice: know your skin type and be aware of the sun's strength in your holiday location.*

*Therefore, until labelling and testing is uniform worldwide, use SPFs and Factor numbers as approximate guides only to the protective value of a product. A dermatologist's advice: know your skin type and be aware of the sun's strength in your holiday location. That's more important than SPF ratings.*

**B**ase time for your skin type to sun without protection (never recommended). Remember to account for factors such as location, the time of day and your surroundings: fair skins, maximum of just 10 minutes between 11 am and 3 pm in the heat, rising to 20 minutes for very dark skins, during the first days of exposure.

## SENSUAL SHADES FOR SUMMER TANNING

The great thing about making up tanned skin is that you need very little. Your three top options:

✳ Coral and shell pink are pretty for eyes and lips on the beach. Aim for a 'barely there' hint of colour, especially on lightly tanned skin. Treat your mouth to a lipstick with moisturizing and sunscreening ingredients.

✳ Gold and copper on lips *and* eyes, plus a hint of bronzing face powder for shimmering nights are exotic and tan-enhancing.

✳ Flash a brilliant hue of liner across your top lid and pick a sheer tint of hothouse fuchsia or sunny orange lip colour for tropical beauty in an instant.

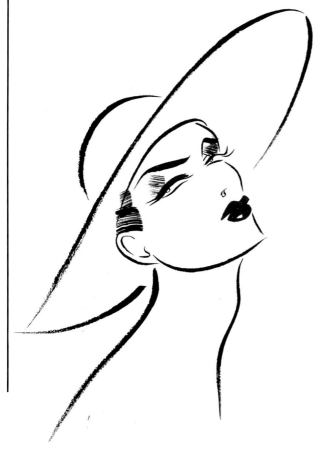

# your tan plan

Take special care during the first few days of exposure to the sun, even if you already have a tan or tan easily. The production of melanin (protective pigmentation of the skin) takes 3 days to build up to its optimum functioning level. For initial exposure dermatologists recommend sunscreens with a high SPF, preferably 15 (SPF 15 is adequate for most sun-tanning).

*Pick the formulation suited to your skin type. If you have oily or acne-prone skin, look for a non-greasy gel or oil-free lotion. If you have normal to dry skin, try a cream or milky lotion. Many of the more recent products on the market are longer-lasting, water-resistant formulae.*

Apply sunscreen before putting on your swimsuit so that you don't miss the skin along your tan line.

## FIND YOUR SKIN TYPE AND TIME YOUR SUN EXPOSURE!

| Classification | Reaction to sun | Examples | Natural protection time* | Recommended SPF for first 2/3 days |
|---|---|---|---|---|
| **I)** Sensitive | Always burns easily Never tans | Red-haired Freckled | 10 minutes | 10+ High to ultra-high |
| **II)** Sensitive | Always burns easily Tans minimally | Fair skinned Blue eyed | 10–15 minutes | 10+ High to ultra-high |
| **III)** Normal | Burns moderately Tans gradually | Darker Caucasian | 20 minutes | 8–10 Moderate to high |
| **IV)** Normal | Burns minimally Tans always | Mediterranean | 20–30 minutes | 6–8 Moderate |
| **V)** Insensitive | Rarely burns Tans profusely | Middle Eastern Latin American | High | 4 Low |
| **VI)** Insensitive | Rarely burns Deeply pigmented | Negroes | Excellent | 2 Low |

Step down to a lower factor – for example, from SPF10+ to SPF8 – after a few days if your skin is not red or tender, stay on the lower protection for a few days and then move down again. Because there are no international standards for determining the sun protection factor of sunscreens, it is best to think in terms of ultra-high, high, medium and low protection.

*Natural protection time: exposure to sun between 11 am and 3 pm without burning

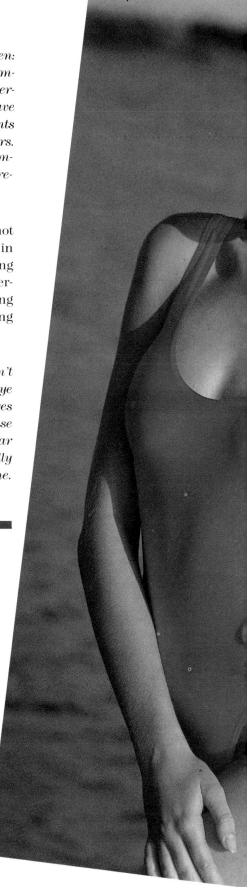

# ZEST

Your tan plan continued

**Re**-apply sun protection often: every 80 minutes or after swimming or perspiring heavily. Super-waterproof brands which have secret waterproofing ingredients are claimed to stay put for hours. However, dermatologists recommend sticking to the 80 minute re-application rule.

---

**Re**-applying sunscreen does not increase the time you can stay in the sun. For instance, applying SPF8 will give a fair-skinned person around 80 minutes of tanning time before they burn. Re-applying the screen doesn't extend this.

---

**T**ake care of eyes and lips: don't use regular sunscreens in the eye area. They may run into the eyes and provoke sensitivity, cause puffiness and even block tear ducts. Choose a block specifically designed for this delicate zone.

*Playing beach games or walking along the water's edge will mean less chance of burning from concentration of the sun's rays on the same skin zone.*

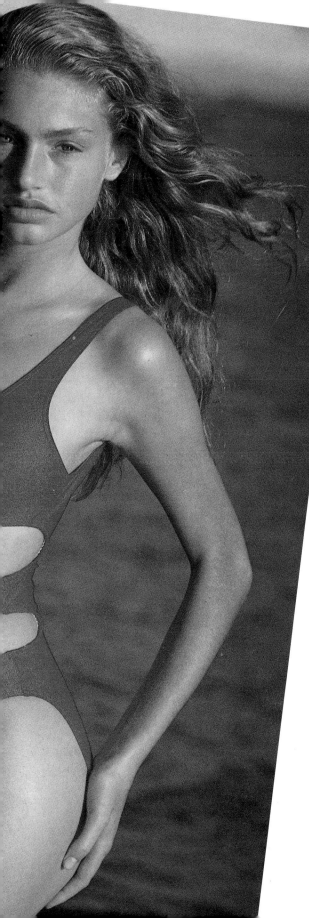

*Waxy lip blocks are not suitable for the eyes unless the product states to the contrary. Lips have no melanin and need protecting with a high-factor waxy stick formulated for lips or with coloured zinc oxide block.*

## BEACH FUN

Playing beach games or walking along the water's edge will mean less chance of burning from concentration of the sun's rays on the same skin zone – and no chance of falling asleep! Watch out for rising body temperature, dehydration and heat stroke.

**SUMMER ZEST**

## FACE AND BODY SAVERS

**R**esist the temptation to get too brown on your face, where the toll of sunbathing will surely show. Scientists believe that 99% of wrinkles are caused by sunbathing. Invest in a 'total block' or high-protection product. Many are now specifically developed for the face with added skin-soothing and moisturizing ingredients. Always wear a good pair of sunglasses (see page 81).

✳ **Fake it:** investigate the instant colour boost of bronzing gel or powders for your face or the longer-term effects of fake tanning for the body. Fake tanning products contain dihydroxy-acetone (DHA) which reacts with proteins in the skin to produce a tan-like tint.

Create a sun-kissed look sans sun with these simple hints designed to side-step blotches and streaks:

✳ Use water-based lotion or gel for oily skins; a powder or cream for normal or dry skins. But if your skin is dry or lined, check that a gleaming powder doesn't emphasize wrinkles. Remember, the paler your skin, the more artificial the results will look.

✳ Always apply your tanning cream or powder to very clean, smooth – recently exfoliated – skin that has been thoroughly dried so that the colour doesn't grab on to dry skin areas. Don't use fake tan immediately after shaving or waxing as this will irritate the skin. Soften dry areas like knees, heels and elbows with a little body lotion beforehand.

✳ Use a cosmetic sponge, or a puff for powder, and sweep the fake tanning product on with long strokes. Don't rub. Avoid the eyes, eyebrows and hairline.

✳ Using a sponge avoids hand-staining – but if you have used your hands, wash carefully immediately after application, especially around the nails.

✳ Wait an hour before dressing or going to bed after applying fake tan.

✳ Fake tans don't give you any protection so apply your regular sunscreen too.

✳ Don't wash skin for at least 3 hours after application. But do

---

## KEEP YOUR TAN GLOWING LONGER

✳ Shower off salt water or chlorine immediately after swimming to prevent skin dehydration.

✳ Use the gentlest cleansing shower or bath gels (not soaps) to avoid drying the skin further.

✳ Slough off dead surface skin cells regularly while you're on holiday and afterwards, when you've stopped sunbathing. Contrary to wearing away your tan, exfoliating lets a golden colour glow through and allows moisturizers to penetrate.

✳ Always apply moisturizer after sun exposure to soothe and hydrate. Slap on to damp skin to seal extra moisture in. Move quickly – a dry atmosphere will start to steal your skin's own moisture after a few minutes.

cleanse thoroughly later on, as usual.

✳ A fake tan starts to fade in a few days as skin cells slough off.

## CAN YOU ACCELERATE A TAN?

Ingredients such as tyrosine, an amino acid that occurs naturally in the body, are now being included in 'pre-tan accelerators' and in many suntanning preparations. Manufacturers claim that if you apply the pre-tanners several days before exposure to sun, they will kick off melanin production so that when you hit the beach you'll tan faster. But do they work? Some scientists are sceptical about their efficacy. We can only await the results of long-term research on the subject.

If you have used a pre-tan accelerator, or are using sun-screening preparations with tan boosting ingredients, don't be tempted to stay out baking for longer – you're still vulnerable to burning and sun-damage and need to take your skin type into account and apply your regular SPF product.

## REPAIRING THE DAMAGE

A recent scientific study has found that, when protected from further onslaughts of the sun, damaged skin does repair itself.

However, UVA rays surround us constantly. They are relatively strong even during times such as morning and late afternoon when the burning UVBs are fairly weak. They pass through windows and pulse from almost every light source. Invest, therefore, in a moisturizer that contains UVA/UVB screens for year-round wear and remember to take it down on to your neck and chest when you're wearing a low-cut top (lines and pigmentation marks on the delicate chest skin are instantly 'ageing') and apply to hands. Eye shadows and lipsticks with UV filters are now being introduced for everyday use.

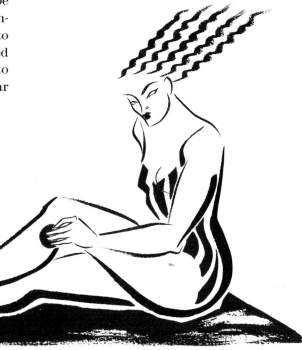

SUMMER ZEST

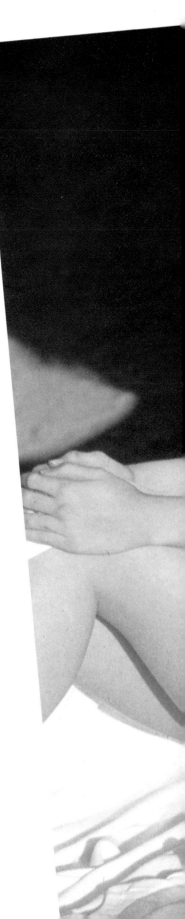

## SOLAR POWER

Many factors affect the intensity of UV light.

✳ Radiation is strongest around midday, when sunlight travels vertically through the ozone layer. Don't sunbathe between 11 am and 3 pm, particularly until natural melanin production increases (about 3 days). Because of the scatter effect of sunlight by molecules in the atmosphere, it is possible to burn even in the shade at midday.

✳ UV radiation passes through clouds.

✳ Altitude increases the strength of UVB rays. In general, every 300 m (1000 ft) above sea level adds 4% to the burning effect of sunlight.

✳ Reflection is another factor that ups solar power. White surfaces, snow, water and sand all reflect UV rays; 40% of direct sunlight can penetrate water to a depth of 5 m (16 ft) and burn skin, even while swimming.

✳ Consider the season: at the equator it is always high summer.

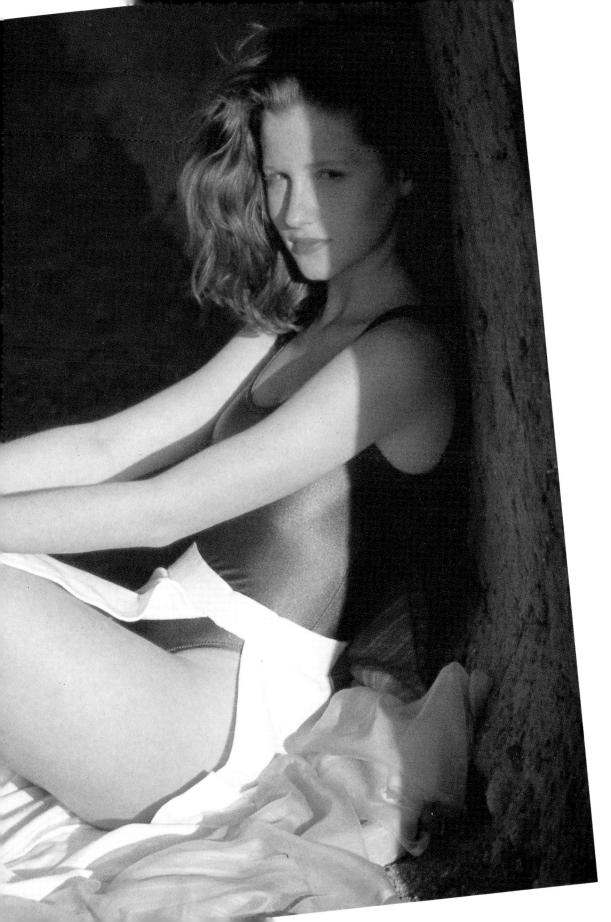

# Skin cancer

Twice as many women as men get skin cancer. Those most often affected are fair-skinned people who spend a lot of time in the sun, and it has also been associated with sunburn in childhood and short, sharp bursts of sun exposure to unprotected skin. Today, with the earth's protective ozone layer being increasingly destroyed by chemicals, particularly chloroflurocarbons, (CFCs), the occurrence of skin cancer may be set for a dramatic increase. In addition, new research has shown that UVB radiation is linked to a weakening of the immune system.

There are several types of skin cancer. The most dangerous, malignant melanoma, is strongly associated with sudden, short sharp exposures to sunlight by those of us who normally have our skin covered. Malignant melanomas can develop from pigment cells in a mole, or from pigment cells in ordinary skin which undergo a change (see below) – usually producing a lesion or lump in the skin. Basal cell and squamous cell cancers are the most common and least harmful forms of skin cancers; they appear as lumps or lesions which may grow slowly and ulcerate. Squamous cell carcinoma may spread to other parts of the body late in their course. Basal cell carcinoma spreads locally. It becomes more difficult to remove as it gets bigger. Squamous cell carcinoma is more aggressive, but has a 95% cure rate. Malignant melanomas spread rapidly; there is approximately a 40% five-year survival rate. Malignant melanoma occurs on areas that are exposed to sunlight. Common sites are the legs and the back.

It's vital that skin cancer, particularly malignant melanoma, is treated in the early stages. Any change in existing moles or the appearance of new wart-like growths should be examined by a doctor. Check regularly for irregularity in the surface or the shape of existing moles, don't wait for discomfort.

*Twice as many women as men get skin cancer. Those most often affected are fair-skinned people who spend a lot of time in the sun.*

**Watch for the following symptoms:**

**Itching:** *Early malignant melanoma is frequently itchy but not painful. An ordinary mole is neither itchy nor painful.*

**Changes in size:** *Early malignant melanomas grow. Ordinary moles in adults do not grow.*

**Shape:** *Early malignant melanomas have an irregular shape with a ragged outline, unlike ordinary moles, which have a regular outline.*

**Colour:** *Early malignant melanomas usually have a mixture of different shades of brown and black so the colour is very irregular. Ordinary moles may be dark brown or black but are all one shade.*

**Redness/inflammation:** *Many early malignant melanomas are inflamed or have a reddish edge.*

**Bleeding, oozing or crusting:** *Some early melanomas may show one or more of these symptoms and may stick to clothing.*

**Note these sun-provoked skin cancer facts:**

✳ *Using an SPF15 in the first 18 years of life lowers skin cancer odds dramatically.*

✳ *Wearing a bikini carries a 13 times higher risk of developing skin cancer than wearing a one-piece swimsuit. Even sporting a low-backed one-piece increases your risk to 4 times that of wearing a high-back version.*

✳ *UVA rays, as well as the burning UVB rays, are implicated as a cause of skin cancer. The message is: don't use sun beds. (UVA rays are also believed to be wrinkle-promoting, reaching deeper into the dermis than the UVB rays. Approximately one-third of people using sun beds do not obtain a tan.) If you do use a sun bed, remember that you still need adequate sunscreening protection when you hit the beach.*

*Using an SPF15 in the first 18 years of life lowers skin cancer odds dramatically.*

# hair care in the sun

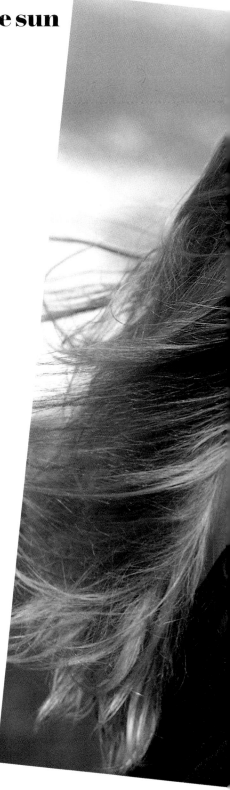

Sun, chlorine, salt water and salty breezes can wreak havoc on your hair. Exposing unprotected hair to these summer elements bleaches and discolours it, and dehydrates and weakens the hair's structure, causing it to break. If your hair has been chemically treated it will be more porous and at special risk. For example, bleached hair may become green-tinged by algae-control chemicals used in pools. Before going away anywhere hot, check with your hairdresser how your colour or perm will stand up to the drying effects of the sun.

Use these solutions to keep your hair healthy and lustrous through steamy, summer days.

✳ Wear a loose-fitting scarf or hat.

✳ Use a protective hair shield with UV screens – usually in gel formula, they give hair a glossy sheen too. Another good tip is to braid hair, or tie it into a ponytail or topknot – this will reduce the surface area subjected to sunlight.

*Summer elements can be harsh on your hair. Take your pick from the latest hair protection tactics and keep your hair gleaming.*

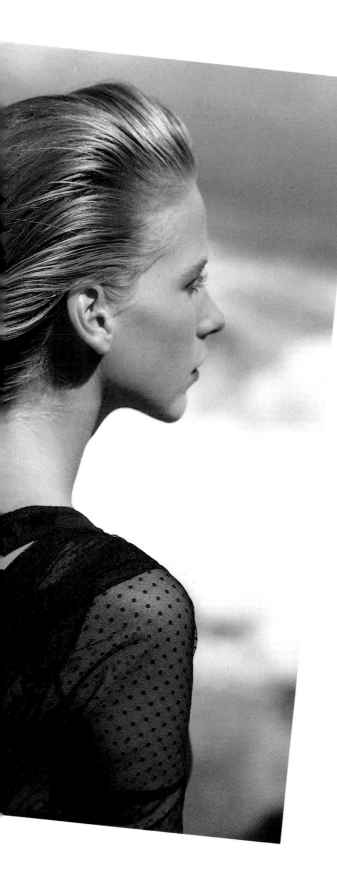

✳ Don't apply oil to hair that's having a sunning session – it attracts the sun's rays and 'fries' the hair, speeding damage.

✳ Some mousses and hairsprays now contain UV screens. They won't give enough coverage for day-long protection but are useful for a few hours sightseeing.

✳ Protect hair from salt and chlorine when swimming with a hair sunscreen or, if you don't have one, a heavy-weight conditioner. Rinse thoroughly with fresh, as opposed to salt water.

✳ Take a deep-conditioning hair mask on holiday with you. If hair is becoming frazzled, use it – just do the ends if they are dry – and tie on a scarf. Alternatively, smooth it on before you take a siesta to re-moisturize and nourish your hair.

✳ Wear a swimming cap to protect bleached hair from chlorine, or turn to p. 113 for the problem-solvers in the Hair Help Clinic. **99**

# **h**ealth action: thrush

This is a common vaginal problem, caused by the yeast fungus candida albicans. This results in inflammation of the vagina which produces redness, swelling, itching and discharge.

### Causes:
*Over-frequent washing. Use of antibiotics or vaginal deodorants which kill natural defences. Pregnancy or the contraceptive pill.*

### Precautions:
✳ Avoid over-frequent washing.

✳ Avoid potential irritants such as scented soaps and bubble baths. Never use disinfectant in your bathwater.

✳ Take care to wipe from the front to the back after a bowel movement.

✳ Cases of continual or recurring thrush have been helped by diet, according to the PMT Advisory Service. (Many PMT symptoms seem to be aggravated by candida.) They recommend avoiding sugary and starchy foods (yeast thrives on them) and foods that are high in yeast, including alcohol, citrus fruit drinks (freshly squeezed juice is yeast-free), bread, cakes etc, malted cereals and drinks, mushrooms, miso, dried fruits, left-over food and vitamins (unless they are labelled yeast free).

✳ Wear loose-fitting cotton underwear and stockings rather than tights.

### Treatment:
✳ Try inserting a little live yogurt into the vagina for 3 days after menstruation.

✳ Adding salt to your bath can help.

✳ Antibiotics may be prescribed but are best avoided because they may destroy the vagina's own beneficial bacteria. Thrush often occurs after a course of antibiotics.

✳ Ensure that your partner is not affected too. He should use a sheath to protect himself and prevent the infection being passed back to you.

✳ Your GP may prescribe medicated creams.

# ZEST AUTUMN

Want to revitalize your body and
mind? Follow this feel-great
guide to autumn and you'll revel
in the pleasure of perfume.
Switch on to the power of
breathing. Take fitness in your
stride. Beat the health-breakers
with essential oils. Get clued up
on vitamins and minerals. Oh,
and don't miss the at-a-glance
hair glossary for the shiniest
hair...

**101**

AUTUMN

ZEST

# b-r-e-a-t-h-e

**B**reathing correctly is something many of us often forget, or don't know how to do. The result: we miss out on its health-giving qualities and our bodies cannot reach their optimum regenerative capacity. We may feel tired for no apparent reason, find it difficult to concentrate over long periods and

*Learn to breathe correctly and energize your body and mind!*

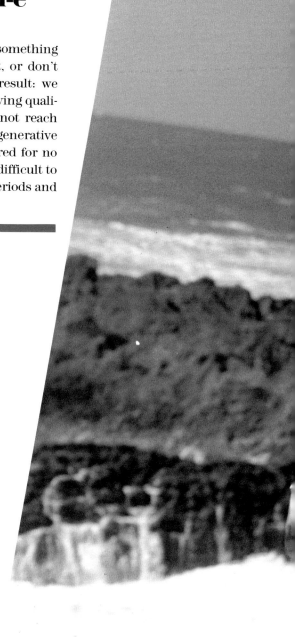

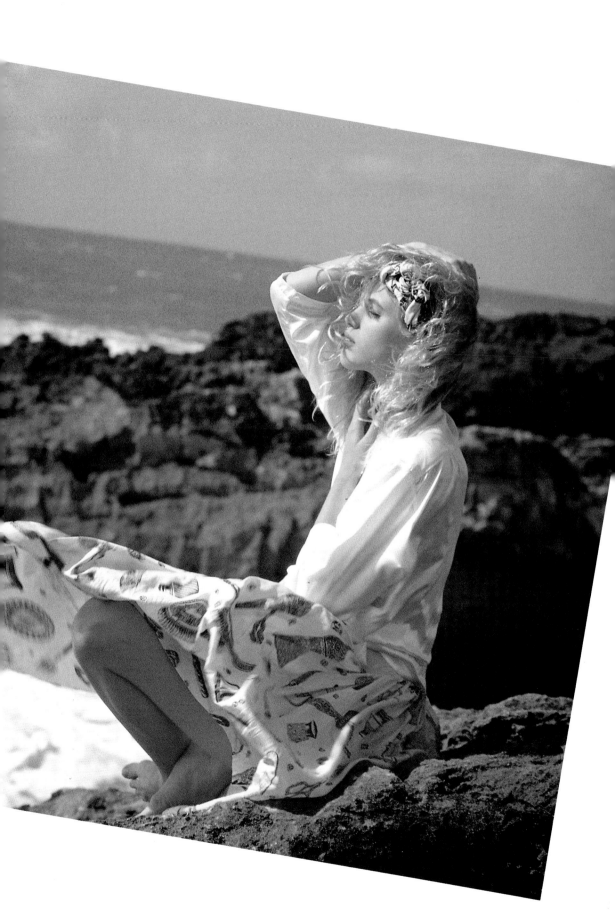

have depleted energy reserves. When we inhale we take in energy-generating oxygen. When we exhale, we remove waste products from our system, particularly carbon dioxide.

Conscious deep breathing will reduce the build-up of toxins in your system, which can occur when you breathe shallowly. It aids digestion by massaging the digestive organs. And it will calm you, clarify your thoughts and increase circulation to the brain, stimulating the production of mood-improving endorphins. Yoga teachers use the revitalizing powers of breathing to simultaneously relax and energize the body and mind – yoga classes are a useful way to learn to breathe correctly and to develop the habit. They recommend inhaling through the nose and exhaling through the mouth.

## THE AIR THAT WE BREATHE

Negative ions are a vital component of fresh air. Smoke, pollution, television and VDU screens, air conditioning and synthetic furnishings all alter the ionic balance. Ionizers are available which feed negative ions back into the air. They also enable negatively charged particles of pollens, dust and smoke to be deposited on to surfaces more readily – with the result that you inhale fewer from the atmosphere.

## *EASY BREATHING EXERCISES:*

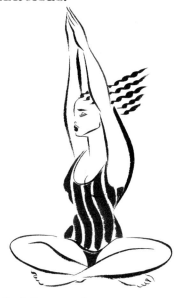

\* ***Quick energizer:*** *Sit with your legs crossed, or in a chair with feet on the floor. Raise hands above head so that upper arms are almost hugging ears, elbows straight, palms together. Inhale through nose as you turn head, body and arms to left. Exhale as you turn to right. Bring arms down slowly, relax shoulders, breathe in, lift arms and repeat again. Do this for 30 seconds. Rest arms and repeat again.*

## GOOD BREATHING TECHNIQUE

To breathe properly, it's important to relax the stomach and solar plexus and to expand the lower back when you inhale. Many women hold their stomachs in to make them look flat and take shallow breaths using the chest, forgetting the diaphragm. When you inhale, the muscles of the abdomen should draw the diaphragm down. We often breathe quickly and in the chest only when we are under stress.

Your posture will affect your ability to breathe for maximum effect. When you're bent over a desk, the chest becomes cramped and the lungs are unable to fill to capacity. Straighten your back (without straining or holding it rigid) and allow your chin to drop forward slightly as you lengthen the back of the neck to free any tension there.

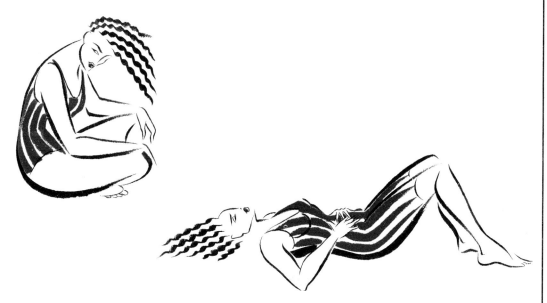

✴ **Helps prevent lower back pain:** Sit with your legs crossed and hold your shins, back stretched up and straight. (You can also do this exercise in a chair with your feet on the floor, hands on knees.) Inhale as you gently press the lower back forward; exhale as you curve spine back. Limit the movement to the lower spine, keep head still and don't rock back and forth. Repetitions: 10–15 daily.

✴ **Deep breathing:** Place hands on stomach with fingertips touching. Relax stomach, exhale to a slow count of 4, hold for 4 and then inhale through the nose. Your abdomen should expand so that the fingertips separate. Exhale, pulling navel in to help complete the exhalation process. Repetitions: 5–10 daily.

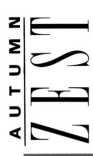

# health action: pre-menstrual tension

From 3 to 14 days before a period you are likely to suffer one or more of 150 symptoms associated with pre-menstrual tension (PMT – also known as Pre-Menstrual Syndrome or PMS). The most common are:

* tension
* anxiety
* irritability
* breast tenderness
* depression
* fatigue
* bloatedness
* cravings for food

Unlike period pains, which often lessen after childbirth, unfortunately PMT frequently worsens.

Studies by the PMT Advisory Service have found that changing your diet can greatly alleviate the symptoms. To help beat PMT they recommend that we:

* Reduce refined carbohydrates (sugar, cakes, biscuits, sugary drinks)
* Limit consumption of dairy products (they affect absorption of magnesium, a mineral that PMT sufferers are frequently deficient in)
* Reduce coffee, tea and alcohol consumption
* Reduce salt
* Eat leafy green vegetables and salads daily
* Eat wholefoods – wholegrains and cereals, fresh fish and some poultry
* Use high quality vegetable oils, such as sunflower or safflower and eat linseeds, sunflower, sesame and pumpkin seeds for the linoleic acid they contain
* Consider taking supplements of vitamin B6 and magnesium. Evening Primrose Oil has proven beneficial
* Cut down on smoking
* Exercise regularly

## HEALTH CHECKLIST

Keep a file detailing your health checks and results. Family history may mean certain tests are done more often, but the dates below are a guide:

*Breast examination*
Examine your breasts every month. Your doctor or family planning clinic should check them once a year. Mammograms should be done approximately every two years after 35.

*Cervical smear*
Under 35, every two years. Over 35, every year (although some doctors believe they should be done every year if you are sexually active).

*Gynaecological examination*
Under 35, every 3 years
Age 35–49, every 2 years
Over 50, every year

*Blood pressure*
Under 50, every 2 years
Over 40, every year
If you are on the pill, every year or whenever you visit your doctor

*Heart and lungs*
As for gynaecological examination

*Urine*
As for gynaecological examination

*Cholesterol*
As for gynaecological examination

*Eyesight*
Every year. Soft contact lens wearers, every 6 months. Glaucoma may be included in a regular sight test – tell the optician if it occurred in your family. It will be routinely tested for after age 40.

*Dental*
Every 6 months

# **W**ater workout

Working out in water is a great way to strengthen and tone muscles, even for non-swimmers. Because you weigh only 10% of your normal weight in water, physical strain on the body is reduced to a minimum. This makes water exercise especially useful if you are underfit, overweight or suffer from joint problems such as weak knees and ankles.

Use a water workout as part of your weekly exercise programme. If you are very unfit, increase repetitions gradually. You should feel energized by pool moves, not exhausted! Always finish your pool workout with a slow bob (see below) or by swimming a few lengths. Seal these pages inside a plastic folder and head for the cool, refreshing and revitalizing benefits of water...

**Bobbing** *is used as a warm-up and between exercises to loosen muscles and keep you warm if the water is chilly. Stand chest-deep in the water and jog on the spot. Because of the resistance of the water you'll find that your movements are slowed down. Hold on to the side of the pool until you've got the hang of it and then bob further out. Use your arms to help keep your balance. Keep bobbing until your body feels warm and you are slightly out of breath.*

Now you are ready to work on specific body zones. These exercises are divided into upper, middle and lower body workouts. Alternate the body area you exercise and bob between each exercise – bob gently or more vigorously for 30 seconds to one minute, depending on how tired you feel.

## Upper body

For upper body exercises always stand with feet comfortably apart and arms submerged.

CHEST AND UPPER BACK: Keeping shoulders down, bring arms out to the sides of body until they are at chest level. With palms flat and facing forwards smoothly sweep arms together in front of chest. Turning palms to face back-wards, push arms back as far as they will naturally go. Repetitions: 4–8 times.

FRONT AND BACK OF ARMS: Arms by sides, palms flat. With palms facing forwards, raise arms smoothly, keeping them straight and parallel. Turn palms down and press arms back as far as they will go. Keep your shoulders down. Repetitions: 4–8 times.

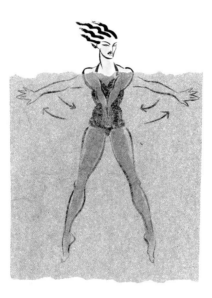

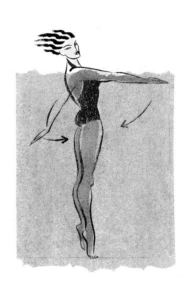

## Middle body

BOTTOM FIRMER: Stand side-ways-on to the pool wall, holding on to side for support. Bend right knee towards chest and straighten leg out in front. Slowly sweep leg back-wards until buttock squeezes, keep-ing back straight. Repetitions: 4–8 times with each leg.

**Note:** Waterproof personal stereos have recently been launched in some countries. A great way to add excitement to your lap swimming and your water workout.

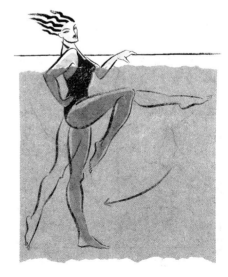

## Lower body

INSIDE/OUTSIDE THIGH: Stand at a diagonal facing slightly away from pool wall. Hold edge rail for support. Lift outer leg to side without tilting body away from lifting leg. Sweep leg forwards, so it crosses in front of the supporting leg. Sweep out again. Repetitions: 4–8 times with each leg.

BODY STRETCH: In the water, face pool wall and hold on to edge rail with both hands. Bend knees and place feet against wall below hands. Slowly extend legs and arms and hold for 30 seconds. Gradually return to starting position and repeat. Make sure your body is really warm when you stretch. The stretch increases the closer your feet are to your hands.

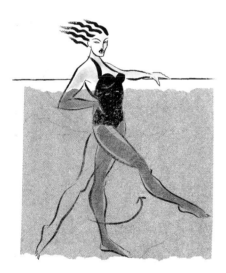

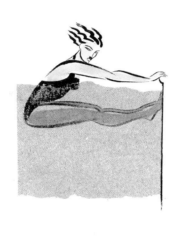

STOMACH-STRENGTHENER: With back against pool wall, rest arms over the edge rail. Keep shoulders down. Pull in stomach muscles so pelvis tilts back and lower back presses up against wall. Then bend right knee and draw it up towards chest. Lower and repeat with other leg. Repetitions: 4–8 times with each leg.

**Note:** To increase the strength of this exercise, raise both legs at the same time pulling in from the stomach. At no time should you feel strain in the lower back.

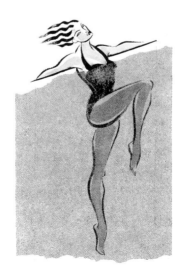

**ZEST**

# fall for fragrance

**I**ntoxicating, evocative, image-creating, a purely personal pleasure or a potent statement of personality and style. Fragrance can play many parts. Just as you change your clothes with the seasons, so you can change your scent, your very presence.

Many women and men are fascinated by fragrance and have a 'wardrobe' of favourite scents from different perfume families, using them according to the season, occasion, the time of day or their mood.

Fragrance fiends often scent their surroundings, too. One fashion editor sprays Dali into his bathroom when he leaves for work in the morning, so that when he returns it has dissipated to a marvellous smell. A managing director sprays the pillows with her man's fragrance when he's away! And a French perfumier sells absorbent perfumed pebbles in her shops and puts them between the floorboards and into the corners of her home.

*Just as you change your clothes with the seasons, so you can change your scent, your very presence.*

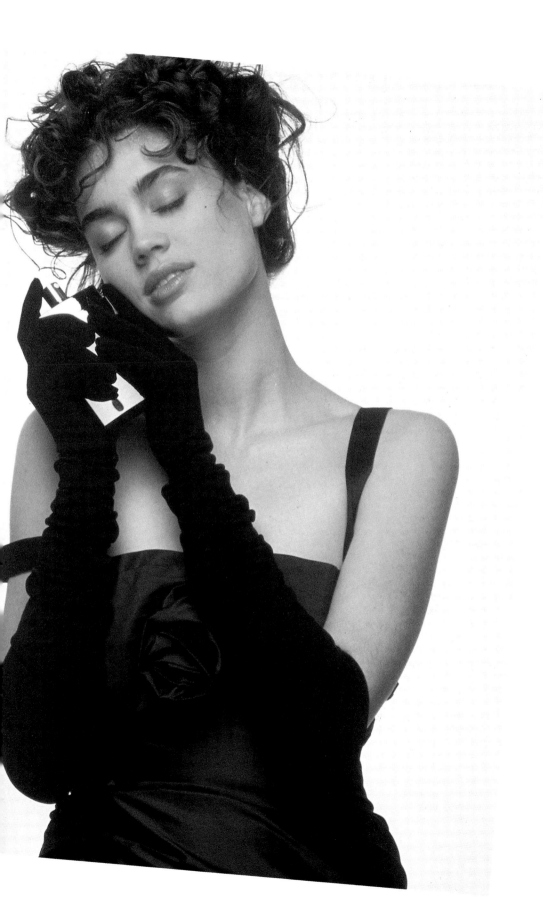

# AUTUMN ZEST

As autumn approaches, you could switch from summer's lightweight citrus, floral and herb scents – so appealing when you want something that goes on icy-cool such as Diorissimo, Hermès', Amazone – to warmer woody notes, such as the chypre family with its wonderfully mossy aroma reminiscent of damp woods and ferns, produced by ingredients such as oakmoss, amber and bergamot. Fragrances such as Femme by Rochas, Guerlain's Mitsouko, and Miss Dior all have the characteristic rich, vital and lasting aura of chypre perfumes.

Seductive, sweet and spicy, the orientals are a heady, sensual choice for the autumn/winter season. A fragrance belonging to the oriental family may also have citrus and floral notes (known as a floral-oriental), with notes, for instance, of ambergris, sandalwood, vanilla, musk and exotic blooms such as ylang ylang and mimosa. Fragrances such as Shalimar and Jicky by Guerlain, Dior's Poison, Youth Dew by Estee Lauder and of course Opium by Yves Saint Laurent have oriental elements.

## CHOOSING A SCENT

*When choosing a perfume, try up to 3 fragrances at a time. Don't smell scent straight from the bottle – you'll just get the initial top note – but apply to the wrist or pulse points, and allow some time for it to 'dry down'. Built up of a harmony of notes, the top notes of perfume are perceived at the beginning of evaporation and are not lasting; the middle notes interact with the natural chemicals in your skin and are the body of the fragrance; the base notes are the foundation of the fragrance and are the longest-lasting.*

## APPLYING FRAGRANCE

As well as the pulse points, freshly washed hair is a good fragrance carrier. Layering your fragrance keeps it subtle and makes it last: starting in the morning with perfumed shower gel and perhaps scented body lotion, you can revive it later with eau de toilette, and save the perfume for the evening.

*A sensuous place to apply scent:* down the centre of your body, from the neck to the waist. Fragrance lasts particularly well on skin underneath clothing.

# hair help clinic

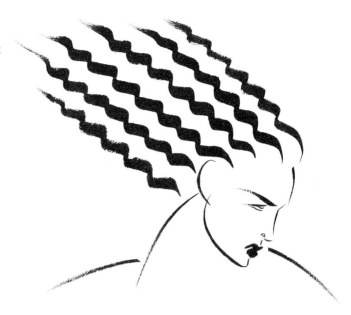

So you want healthy, hi-gloss hair? Fabulous-looking locks come from a gentle hair care regime that's tailored to your hair type and style. And from putting problem-solvers into action immediately, not weeks or months later! Here's how to give your hair the best possible treatment.

## FINE OR LIMP HAIR

### Possible causes:
Heredity. Using a conditioner that is too heavy. Insufficient rinsing.

### Solutions:
✳ Use cleansing and conditioning products formulated for fine hair – avoid lanolin-based products which are too heavy.

✳ Condition ends only.

✳ Use lightweight styling products such as mousse which adds body but avoid gel, pomade and grease. Spray hairspray on to a brush first, rather than directly on to the hair, so that you don't overload the hair.

✳ Too much length can 'thin hair' – the weight makes it drag. A short, blunt cut gives body.

✳ **Perming**: if you don't want the commitment of an all-over perm, a root perm will give style support. Any chemical process – perming, colouring, bleaching – will swell the hair shaft and give the hair added volume and texture provided your hair is in good enough condition. Consult a hairdresser first: the strength of the solutions and techniques used are all-important. Remember that gentle handling of your hair is a vital protective strategy. Chemically treated hair is especially vulnerable to break-age when wet.

✳ Colour can be applied to 'paint the cut', adding emphasis to hair shape.

✳ Style hair in the morning and then try not to touch it again.

**113** ▶

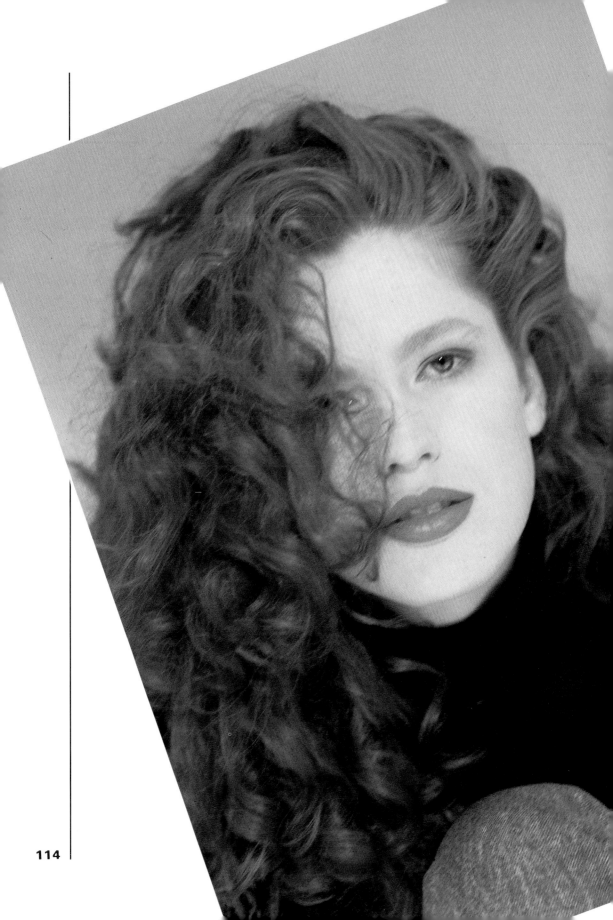

## DULL HAIR

### Possible causes:

Shampoo/conditioner not rinsed out properly. Build-up of residue from hair products. Damage from sun, heated drying/styling tools, chemical treatments. Incorrect drying techniques. Stress.

### Solutions:

✳ Bust 'build-up' by rinsing with a weak solution of white vinegar in water – 30 ml (2 tbsp) to 1.2 litres (2 pints) water – after shampooing and before conditioning. Or use a shampoo specifically formulated for this purpose.

✳ Use a light conditioner formulated for everyday use.

✳ Try a spray glaze product to boost shine (but not on fine hair).

✳ Correct drying keeps the cuticle flat, thereby reflecting the light (for this to happen the layers which make up the cuticle must lie in a downwards direction). Towel-dry by blotting, not rubbing. Use the professionals' blow-drying technique: dry hair section by section using clips. Hold the hairdryer 20 cm (8 inches) or more away, pointing it down the hair shaft, on a low heat setting. Keep the hairdryer moving. For straight hair use a brush with a flat base, for curly hair or waved hair use a round brush.

✳ Charge up with colour. 'Transparent' colours look contemporary and give a lustrous finish. Adding lighter tones makes hair appear brighter and shinier. But remember to keep colour-treated hair clean – oil, dirt, setting aids and sprays can make it look dull, the colour look 'off'.

✳ Eat food sources rich in the B-complex vitamins – green and yellow vegetables, milk, yogurt, eggs, wholegrains.

## DRY HAIR

**Possible causes:**

Heredity. Incorrect or over-frequent use of heated appliances. Chemical treatments such as perms, straighteners, bleaches. Chlorine in swimming pools. Exposure to sun, salt, water, wind. Moisture loss from friction (combing, brushing).

**Solutions:**

✳ Use products formulated for dry hair and deep-condition weekly. Consider investing in a salon deep-conditioning treatment which may use heat to increase the action.

✳ Let hair dry naturally or blow-dry on a low speed and cool setting. Don't attempt to dry dripping-wet hair with a hairdryer – heat damage will be almost guaranteed. Blot dry with a towel first.

✳ Beware of using chemical treatments, especially home perms – your hair could be at 'breaking point', a hair condition where further stress could seriously damage it. Ask the advice of a hair salon.

✳ In the pool, wear a swimming cap. Shampoo thoroughly after swimming and then condition.

✳ Wear a hat or scarf outdoors, or use a protective hair gel with UV screens.

✳ Check that your styling products, such as mousse, do not contain alcohol, which can dry the hair further.

## OILY HAIR

**Possible causes:**

Heredity. Too little washing or over-frequent washing with a harsh product. Over-hot styling products, over-hot water when washing, or over-brushing, which stimulate oil glands.

**Solutions:**

✳ If you wash your hair often, choose a mild shampoo. Shampoos formulated for frequent use are gentle.

✳ You may have a greasy scalp and dry ends – use a mild shampoo at the roots and condition hair carefully at the ends.

✳ Use a comb rather than a brush.

✳ Don't style or touch hair more than necessary.

**Possible causes:**
Effect of humidity on curly or porous hair. Split ends caused by over-vigorous towel-drying, over-drying, brushing too hard or too often or with a brush with rough-edged bristles, back-combing, tugging at tangles. Perming techniques.

**Solutions:**

✳ Have damaged hair cut. Hair cut to one length rather than layered is easier to control.

✳ Don't perm hair immediately before travelling to a hot, humid area. Ideally, allow about 4 weeks for the perm to settle down. (Be careful, too, after exposure to sun when hair may be drier.)

✳ If hair is medium-length or long, use rollers or a round brush when drying to control and smooth the frizz.

✳ Check your hair is completely dry before going out.

✳ Use a cream rinse after every shampoo to control static.

✳ Use mousse or gel to style hair.

✳ Avoid bristle brushes – use plastic-pronged brushes and wide-toothed combs instead.

✳ Use a hairspray to hold and protect against humidity.

✳ Give your hair a deep-conditioning treatment.

✳ Don't brush permed hair.

**Possible cause:**
Blonde hair discoloured by the algae-control chemicals added to chlorinated pool water.

**Solutions:**

✳ A very difficult problem to resolve. Prevention is best so wear a swimming cap.

✳ Rinse with fresh water after swimming and shampoo and condition.

✳ A hairdresser may suggest adding warm, red tones to counteract the green, but this is not always successful.

✳ The green tone may fade with time. Otherwise it can be cut out or you can wait for your hair to grow.

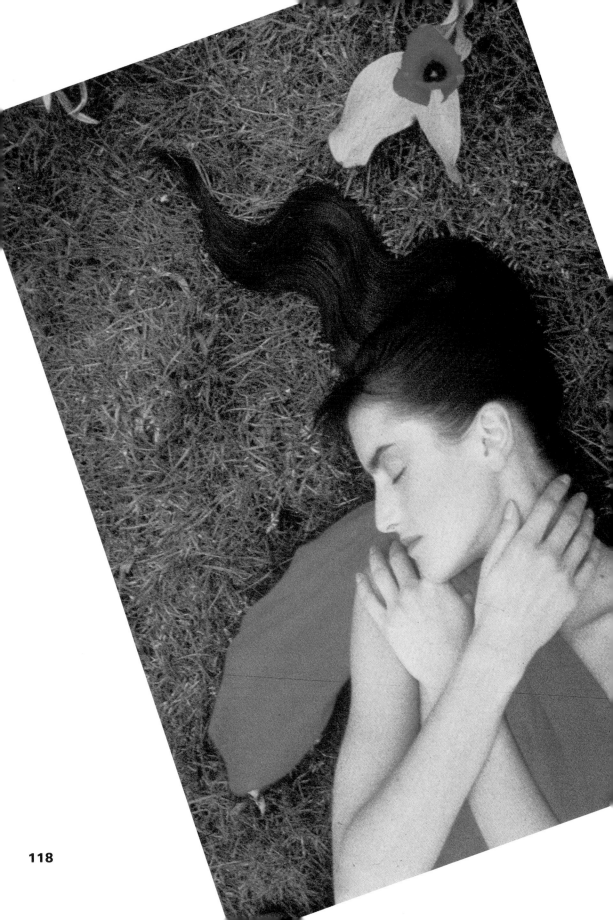

## THINNING HAIR/HAIR LOSS

### Possible causes:

Heredity. Stress. Pulling hair while brushing. Hormonal changes due to ageing, pregnancy, childbirth, menopause or certain metabolic conditions. Poor diet.

### Solutions:

✳ In tests, hormone treatment has proved successful for hereditary hair loss.

✳ Use a conditioner to thicken hair shafts.

✳ Consult your doctor or a trichologist.

✳ Wash hair and massage scalp daily after childbirth.

✳ Eat 12 mg iron and 54 g (2 oz) protein a day.

## FLAKY SCALP

### Possible causes:

Microbes. Hormonal irregularities. A flaky scalp can be caused by infrequent shampooing; inadequate rinsing; sunburnt scalp; stress; incorrect diet.

### Solutions:

✳ Shampoo frequently. 'Dandruff shampoos containing zinc pyrithone are definitely useful,' says Glenn Lyons at the Philip Kingsley Trichology Clinic in London. They should be used for non-inflammatory scalp conditions (an inflamed scalp will be red). Don't use them when the scalp has been cut or scratched. One disadvantage: they can dry the hair.

✳ A flaky scalp that feels tight is probably triggered by stress. Give yourself a scalp massage.

*Fabulous-looking locks come from a gentle hair care regime that's tailored to your hair type and style.*

## YOUR AT-A-GLANCE HAIR GLOSSARY
### Which products will help you achieve first-class style.

**Gel:** A heavy-weight styling product that can be used to create slick, structured styles or as a strong setting lotion, for example, for blow-drying curly hair straight.

**Mousse:** A lightweight styling aid which gives body and texture to the hair. Great for injecting life into fine or limp hair.

You find mousse doesn't work for you? Chances are that you are using too much or not enough. Unfortunately, there are no hard-and-fast rules about this. It's simply a question of trial-and-error, and continuing to experi-ment until you get it right. Hair may feel sticky if you apply mousse when hair is dry or 'crispy' if you apply to damp hair and then leave it to dry without working with it sufficiently. Applied to hair that is too wet the mousse will be diluted and so ineffective. Towel-dry hair, apply mousse and work through the length of the hair with the hands. If mousse has made your hair feel heavy and look dull by the end of the day, simply spritz with water and re-style. This method works with some sculpting lotions too.

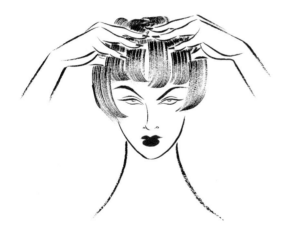

Starting at the front of the head, spread your fingers apart and rest the pads against the scalp. Keeping your fingers in one place, pull and push them apart in a kneading motion. Massage for a minute or more in one area. Move over the head down to the neck and repeat if you like.

### SCALP MASSAGE

Encourage strong, healthy hair growth by giving yourself a once-a-week scalp massage (or as often as daily if you can squeeze it into your schedule), ideally before you wash your hair. Massage stimulates circulation, bringing nutrients, oxygen and hormones to the hair follicles. It is particularly important to help relax you when your scalp feels tight and when you're anxious. Don't massage if the scalp is red and inflamed or if there is any broken skin.

*On these pages, discover how to make the most of hair styling products, relax with a scalp massage and trim your fringe.*

**Pomade/grease:** Both contain some wax, and are very similar in the effects they produce. Use just a touch to give sheen, control and separation. Great for dark and black hair. They can be difficult to wash out.

**Shaping sprays, sculpting lotions:** They help you mould a style and give it staying power; directional sprays can be used to give added body at the roots, or on the ends of the hair to give a short style separation. Follow directions on the product. Some are designed for use on dry, some on wet, hair.

## CUT YOUR OWN FRINGE:

Your best bet for a fringe: have it cut professionally first. It's simple to maintain it from there. Hairdresser Christine Trotter advises: cut on dry hair – hair stretches when it is wet making it more difficult to judge length. Hold the hair between index and middle finger, starting with index finger placed at the bridge of the nose for a fringe that skims the eyebrows. Cut beneath this, a little at a time so that you don't make it too short or take large chunks out. Avoid pulling the hair down too firmly as you cut, which will also alter the length. Feathery fringes can be tricky and, ideally, are best dealt with by a hairdresser.

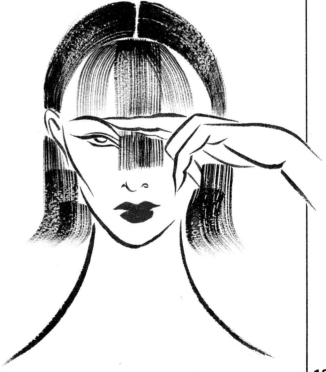

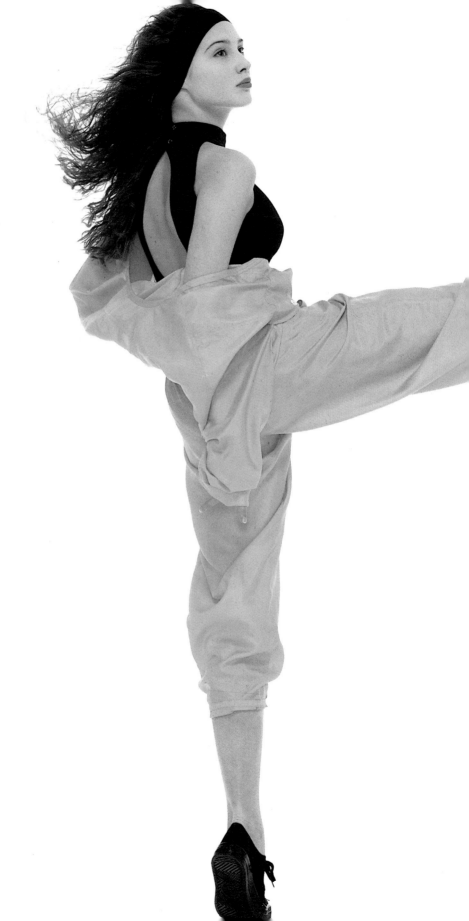

# h ealth action: back care

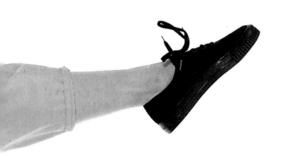

**B**ack pain affects 4 out of 5 people at some time in their lives. Most back pain is muscular and discs rupture as a result of sudden or repetitive strain. Bad posture, bending and lifting incorrectly all contribute to creating back problems.

✴ Women run a greatly increased risk of injuring their backs 3 days before a period. Progesterone levels drop before menstruation, resulting in softer muscles and ligaments which are more susceptible to strains. Take care when doing everyday actions such as bending down to pick something up, or exercising; muscle pulls can even occur when sneezing or coughing.

✴ In addition to carrying extra weight when pregnant, the body produces a hormone which softens ligaments so that the pelvis can expand for the birth. All the ligaments in the body soften so be extra aware of your back's vulnerability during pregnancy.

✴ Sex can be a source of backache. Choose comfortable positions.

*Back pain affects 4 out of 5 people at some time. Keep your back trouble-free with these pointers.* ▶

4/.

* Exercise strengthens the back and is an excellent preventive measure. Choose low-impact aerobic activities if you suspect your back may have weak spots. Exercise is not a solution for backache.

### CHECK YOUR POSTURE:

*The ideal standing position is with a relatively hollow back, stomach and rear tucked in – not poker-backed. Don't try to tuck your bottom in by tilting your pelvis forwards; instead, tighten the buttock muscles.*

### CORRECT SEATING:

Pressure on the spine is least when lying down and greatest when seated. A correct and comfortable chair should have:

* Good lumbar (lower back) support.

* Space in the chair so buttocks can be moved back, allowing the hollow of the back to fit snugly against the lumbar support area.

*The ideal standing position is with a relatively hollow back, stomach and rear tucked in – not poker-backed. Tuck your bottom in by tightening the buttock muscles.*

* Gentle convex curve from the back of the seat to a dipped front, to put as little pressure as possible on backs of knees.

* Softer sections in the seat area to accommodate the bony bit of your bottom where the majority of weight rests.

* Suitable height adjustment.

Lumbar supports, made of foam and looped over the back of a chair, improve poor seating. Some orthopaedic specialists believe that posture-conscious chairs – the sort you kneel into – are suited mostly to young people with no hip or knee problems.

The *way* you sit is important too. Legs should be forward to minimize pressure behind the knee; your knees should be lower than your hips.

### DESK JOBS

Take regular breaks and walk around as much as possible. An ideal work surface should be tilted towards you. VDU screens should be at eye level to avoid placing strain on the neck.

### BENDING DOWN

*Always bend at the knees and not the waist. Keep your back straight, not rounded, holding heavy weights as close to your body as possible.*

### BED TIME

To check the suitability of a bed for you, lie down and insert your hand between the bed and small of your back. The bed is too soft if you cannot do this easily. If your hand slips in and there is plenty of space, the bed is too hard. Your hand should be a snug fit. *When getting out of bed, don't leap up!* Turn on your side, move your legs off the bed and use your arms to push you up to sitting position.

*RELIEVE PAIN*
*Lie down quietly with a hot water bottle against the painful area, in whichever position alleviates the pain (this may be in a foetal position with your knees bent up).*

# grow your own sprouts for super nutrition

In the first few days, the vitamin content of sprouting seeds, beans and pulses increases dramatically. You can buy sprouting trays from health food shops or fix your own at home. Here's how.

*Wash 30 ml (2 tbsp) sprouts in clean water and pick out any pieces of dirt. Leave them to soak in a jam jar for the appropriate time (see right). Throw away the water, then put muslin or a clean tea towel over the top and secure with an elastic band. Rinse by pouring lukewarm water into the jar 2 or 3 times a day, more often in a warm environment. Shake the jar and turn upside down, resting it at an angle to drain. You can get sprouts such as alfalfa to go green by placing them on the windowsill for a day or two, but it is not necessary. When they are ready, place them in a large bowl and cover with water so that you can remove any husks and ungerminated seeds that float. Your sprouts will keep for 4 days in the refrigerator covered.*

**ADUKI BEAN**
Soak: 8–12 hours
Rinse: 3 times a day
Ready: 3–5 days

**ALFALFA**
Soak: 5–8 hours
Rinse: 2–3 times a day
Ready: 5–6 days

**CHICK PEAS**
Soak: 8–15 hours
Rinse: 3 times a day
Ready: 3–4 days

**FENUGREEK**
Soak: 6–8 hours
Rinse: 3 times a day
Ready: 3–4 days

**LENTILS**
Soak: 8–12 hours
Rinse: 3 times a day
Ready: 2–3 days

**MILLET**
Soak: 5–8 hours
Rinse: 3 times a day
Ready: 3–4 days

**MUNG BEANS**
(Bean Sprouts)
Soak: 8–12 hours
Rinse: 4 times a day
Ready: 3–5 days

**WHEAT** (Whole kernel)
Soak: 8–15 hours
Rinse: Twice a day
Ready: 2–3 days

**Note**: You should not sprout kidney beans

# aromatherapy

**T**he ancient art of aromatherapy is a fragrant force today in natural healing. Essential oils extracted from plants and herbs can ease the symptoms of many common ailments such as colds and 'flu, depression and skin problems. Danièle Ryman, one of the world's leading authorities on aromatherapy, explains how you can apply aromatherapeutics to your life.

Aromatics work on two levels. When applied to the skin in combination with a 'carrier oil' during massage, or diluted in our bathwater, the oils, it is believed, penetrate and reach the bloodstream, working on the physiology of our organs and body systems. In addition, the scented molecules have a direct line, via our olfactory receptors, to the emotional centre of the brain. This limbic system is connected to other areas which control the heart rate and blood pressure, breathing patterns, stress reactions and hormones. In studies at Yale University, USA, aromatics have been shown to lower blood pressure and heart rates, to control panic attacks, epilepsy, and pain, and to make people feel calmer, more cheerful and less aggressive.

*Tune in to the scented world of aromatherapy. Use nature's own essential oils to help beat everyday health-breakers, restore vitality and enhance your well-being.*

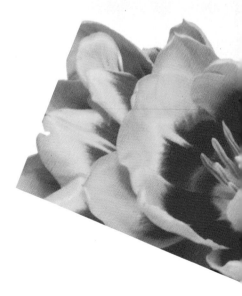

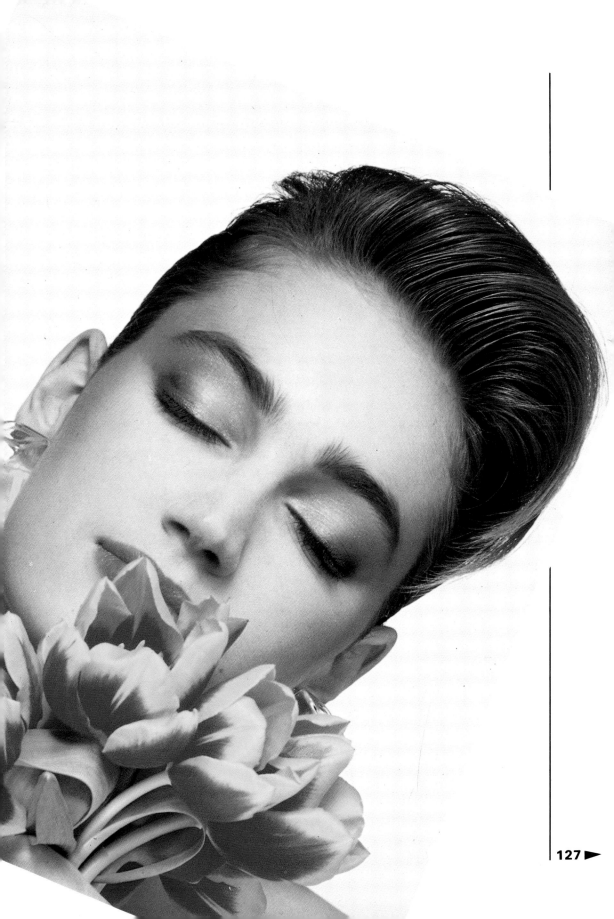

Experienced aromatherapists are able to alleviate many medical conditions, and use their own 'recipes' combining several essential oils to treat individual symptoms.

You can use aromatics at home to relieve the tensions and ills that go hand-in-hand with our contemporary lifestyles. Since some essential oils are anti-bacterial, anti-viral and antiseptic, as well as antibiotic, they can be used to protect us from infection.

Although some natural health enthusiasts may do so, *never* take essential oils internally.

___

Essential oils boost the benefits of massage. Check for allergies before using an oil: place 1 drop inside the elbow or on the wrist and cover with a plaster for a few hours. If a rash develops, you are allergic to the oil. Because aromatherapy oils are concentrated, they are mixed with a carrier oil, such

## AROMATHERAPY OILS TO HELP YOUR HEALTH

**T**he following essential oils may alleviate these everyday health problems:

| | | | |
|---|---|---|---|
| ANXIETY | Neroli | | Cedarwood |
| | | | Eucalyptus |
| | | | Pine |
| | | | Sandalwood |
| ATHLETE'S FOOT | Lemon grass | DEPRESSION | Neroli |
| | | | Rose |
| | | | Ylang ylang |
| BURNS | Lavender (*you can use this neat*) | FATIGUE | *These oils revitalize and stimulate*: |
| | | | Eucalyptus |
| CELLULITE | Cypress | | Geranium |
| | Juniper | | Juniper |
| CIRCULATION | Geranium | | Pine |
| | Lemon | | Rosemary |
| | Orange | | |
| COLDS AND FLU | Cajput, inhaled | HAIR | *Add a few drops to your shampoo*: |
| | Camomile | | |
| | Clove | | |
| | Eucalyptus (*for coughs and catarrh*) | Oily hair | Patchouli |
| | | Dry | Camomile |
| | Lemon | Dull | Lemon |
| | Niaouli | | |
| | Pine | HEADACHE | Camomile |
| CYSTITIS | Cajput | | Lavender |
| | Camomile | | Peppermint |
| | | | Rosemary |

as sunflower or almond. The following proportions are a good general guide: full body massage, 5 drops of essential oil to 20 ml (4 tbsps) of carrier oil; back massage, 2 drops of essential oil to 10 ml (2 tbsps) of carrier oil.

Essential oils can also be used in the bath. Using a pipette, squeeze 10 drops of essential oil under the running tap and swill around in the water before jumping in. Close the door and inhale the uplifting atmosphere.

## Scenting your surroundings:
*Try using essential oils in your home or office during the winter months to protect against colds and flu. Apply a few drops of your chosen oil to a bowl of warm water and place on a radiator. Use a holder designed to fit a light bulb or place a few drops in a plant spray and spritz the room.*

---

| | | | |
|---|---|---|---|
| INFECTIONS (cuts) | Eucalyptus<br>Lavender<br>Sandalwood | Blocked pores<br>Dryness | Rose<br>Camomile<br>Rose |
| INSOMNIA | Basil<br>Camomile<br>Neroli | Eczema | *(Too complicated for self-treatment)* |
| | | Oily tendency | Geranium<br>Juniper |
| MENSTRUAL PROBLEMS | Basil (*helps to regulate menstrual cycle*)<br>Camomile (*for period pains*)<br>Cypress<br>Neroli (*for PMT, feelings of anxiety*) | Puffiness | Rose<br>Sandalwood |
| | | STINGS AND BITES | Camomile<br>Ylang ylang |
| | | STRESS | *Some of the most effective relaxing oils are*:<br>Camomile<br>Lavender<br>Rose |
| MIGRAINE | Basil<br>Camomile<br>Rosemary | | |
| PILES | Camomile<br>Cypress | SUNBURN | Camomile<br>Lavender (*you can apply it neat*) |
| SKIN<br>  Acne | *(Too complicated for self-treatment)* | THRUSH | Lavender |
| | | WATER RETENTION | Rosemary |
|  Allergic skin reactions | Patchouli | | |

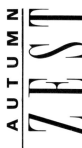
# healthy hand and nail file

### BEST BEAUTY BETS FOR HAND CARE

✳ Often exposed to heat or cold, the hands have relatively few oil glands and so dry faster than other parts of the body. Keep a tube of hand cream next to the sinks at home and in the office.

✳ Unlike the face, hands can't be concealed with cosmetics. Protect them with a sunblock when you're out of doors.

✳ Refine the texture of your hands by gently exfoliating dead cells with a mitt or body scrub, then apply the same moisturizing mask to them as you do to your face when you're treating yourself to a home facial.

✳ Massaging the hands tones the muscles, stimulates circulation and improves skin tone. Apply a massage or aromatherapy oil and, beginning at the fingertips, work over the hands and wrists using circular movements.

✳ When lifting or grabbing objects, keep your fingers as close together as possible to avoid placing the knuckles under undue stress which can weaken the joints and, over a period of time, cause the fingers to spread outwards and look mis-shapen.

✳ Try not to exert force with the hands only – instead, put your body weight, arm and shoulder into opening, twisting or grasping.

**HOW TO HAVE BEAUTIFUL NAILS:** the problem-makers and the simplest solutions.

## RIDGES

CAUSES: Illness. Damage to nail-bed. Heredity. Zinc or calcium deficiencies (which cause horizontal ridges).

TREATMENT:

✳ Once the ridge has formed it is there until the nail has grown out. Buffing will help smooth the surface, but don't do it every day. Or try a three-strength sloughing and buffing file, available from selected chemists and salons.

✳ Use a commercial ridge filler as a base before polish.

✳ See dietary recommendations under White Marks (see page 132).

CAUSES: Nails too dry due to external factors such as detergent, chlorine, sun, wind. Too much soaking in water. Incorrect filing. Nails badly shaped.

TREATMENT:

✳ Moisturize daily with hand or special cuticle cream. Apply moisturizer even when wearing polish to keep cuticles smooth and supple.

✳ Avoid the drying effect of acetone-based polish remover; use one with an oily base instead. Leave polish on for a week, retouching as necessary.

✳ Protect hands during housework by wearing gloves.

✳ Use a nail hardener.

✳ Use a pencil to dial the telephone and knuckle instead of fingertips to push buttons, for example for the lift.

✳ File nails in one direction only – from side to centre using light strokes. Hold the emery board at a 45° angle under the free edge – filing straight up against your nail can make the tip peel. Don't shape nails into a point as filing down the sides will weaken them. After removing polish, wait a few minutes before filing: if the nails aren't completely dry they may split. Don't try to file down very long nails – cut off any excess length with nail scissors or, preferably, clippers. Take small snips, working from one side to the other. Cutting the tip off straight across can weaken your nails.

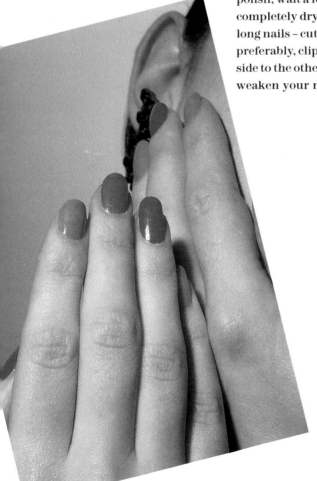

## HANGNAILS

CAUSES: Dry cuticles. Biting and chewing.

TREATMENT:

∗ Daily moisturizing will help keep skin soft.

∗ Push cuticles back with an orange-stick wrapped in cotton wool during home manicure and clip off any hangnails.

∗ Cuticles are hard to keep looking neat and must be handled with care to avoid damaging the growth centre of the nail. Never pull or tear the skin or cut the cuticle itself – once cut, it will grow back a little thicker than before. When you take a bath, push them back gently while still soft with the fingertips.

## YELLOWING

CAUSES: Staining from orange or red nail polishes. Pool chlorine. Nicotine.

TREATMENT:

Soak nails in lemon juice for a few minutes to whiten them.

∗ Some salons offer electric buffing for stain removal. Or use the slougher/buffer designed for ridge smoothing. Both methods should be done very lightly.

∗ Use a base coat under polish and try wearing clear or pale polishes until stain grows out.

## WHITE MARKS

CAUSE: Indication of zinc, not calcium, deficiency.

TREATMENT:

∗ Both zinc and calcium are needed for healthy nails. Your diet should contain 20 mg of zinc (approximately 12 mg from supplements), 800 mg of calcium (approximately 450 mg from supplements). Food sources of both include spinach and Cheddar cheese.

# Walk your way to all-round fitness

Fitness walking is a fast-growing exercise movement. It's easy, energizing, mood-enhancing, stress-relieving and you can do it anytime, anywhere. An all-important plus-point: there's less stress on your joints than with other, higher-intensity workouts like jogging. Although you need to spend longer walking than you would doing, say, an aerobics class, the cardio-vascular (heart and lung) training effect is the same. And, as with any aerobic activity, regular walking boosts your metabolic rate.

∗ *Good footwear. This is really the only thing you need for exercise walking. Your shoes should be comfortable and supportive with cushioning to enhance your natural spring and to help propel you forwards. Specialist shoes are available from good sports shops. For trekking, cross-country, or hill-walking you will need a stouter, water-repellent walking shoe or boot with strong foot and ankle support to help avoid strain. Wear thick socks in natural wool or cotton to absorb sweat. When buying shoes make sure there is plenty of room for thick socks and to allow for natural expansion when your foot is hot.*

∗ *Get ready.* As with all exercise, a little preparation goes a long way. Ease your muscles into readiness by performing some stretches, especially for calves, and fronts and backs of thighs. Check that your body is warm before you stretch – walk up and down the room or footpath for a few minutes.

∗ *Back of thigh*: Stretch right leg straight out in front and rest heel on bench or stair. Bend left leg slightly, rest hands lightly on right leg and lean over keeping back straight until you feel back of right thigh stretch. Hold 10–30 seconds. Repeat with left leg. More stretches next page.

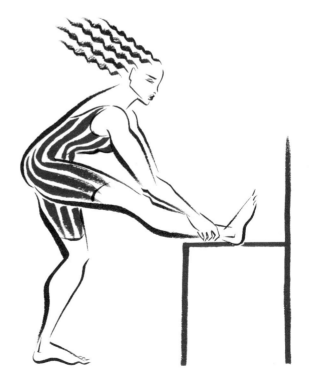

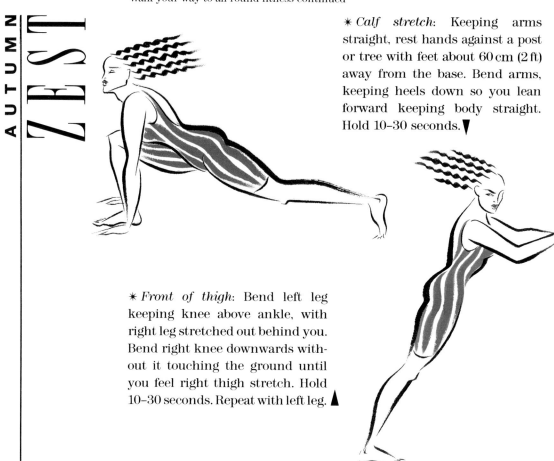

✳ *Calf stretch*: Keeping arms straight, rest hands against a post or tree with feet about 60 cm (2 ft) away from the base. Bend arms, keeping heels down so you lean forward keeping body straight. Hold 10–30 seconds. ▼

✳ *Front of thigh*: Bend left leg keeping knee above ankle, with right leg stretched out behind you. Bend right knee downwards without it touching the ground until you feel right thigh stretch. Hold 10–30 seconds. Repeat with left leg. ▲

Walk gently for the first couple of minutes, taking a few slow deep breaths before you stride out briskly. Slow down again for the last 2 minutes and end your walk with a few more leg stretches. Hold each stretch for 20–30 seconds at this stage, while you are still warm, to increase flexibility.

✳ Walking style. *Always try to walk tall (spine lengthened, shoulders relaxed) – this keeps you moving freely. Step out, putting the heel down first and roll through to push off from the ball of your foot and toes. Keep your leg straight so it sweeps through its full range of movement from the hip. As one leg swings forwards, the opposite arm swings up naturally. Don't try to force any movement and keep your body moving in an easy rhythm. Normal walking firms calves, fronts and backs of thighs; developing a longer stride gives abdominals and buttocks a workout, too.*

✳ *How far to go*: For cardiovascular fitness you are aiming to raise your heart rate to around 65% to 80% of its maximum (to calculate it: 220 beats per minute minus your age, multiplied by the training percentage gives you the rate.) If you're underfit, start at 60% and always go by how you feel. Aim for a walking pace of 5–6.5 km (3–4 miles) per hour, i.e. 1.5 km (1 mile) in 15–20 minutes. If this is hard going at first, build up gradually. When you begin your walking programme, check your pulse rate now and again (keeping your legs moving). You should never be more than comfortably out of breath and should be able to hold a conversation while you walk. If you're totally shattered at the end of your walk you've over-done it.

*Choose the form of walking that you can fit into your lifestyle.*
✳ City walking. *Can take you from home to work and back again, around a park or on a tour of interesting places. But to keep up the momentum of your fitness walking, plan a challenging walk to look forward to and train for.*

✳ Hiking/backpacking. *Plan a route from one of the many maps and books available. Pack some provisions and a lightweight waterproof. Breathe in the fresh country air and feel your mind relax as you stride out through peaceful surroundings. If you are considering serious all-day hikes, you should be able to walk 6.5–8 km (4–5 miles) a day com-fortably.*

✳ Interval walking. *Adds variety to your walking workout. Occasionally walk very quickly for 2 minutes and then slow back to your regular pace. To pick up speed increase both the rate and length of your stride, allowing your arms to swing out freely for balance.*

✳ Trekking. *This involves walking over several days or even weeks and can be done in some of the world's most exotic locations. Make sure you train for a trekking holiday, particularly if it involves high altitudes. Trekking can give you the holiday of a lifetime and the ultimate fitness walk!*

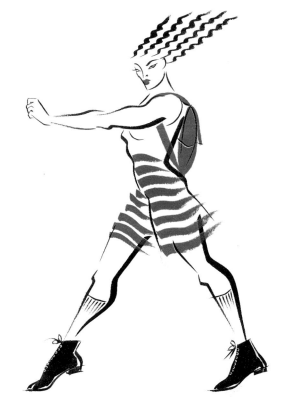

*Walking is easy, energizing, mood-enhancing, stress-relieving and you can do it any time, anywhere.*

# ZEST

# WINTER

Warm to winter with our top-to-toe, health-enhancing hints. Fight fatigue and boost your vitality. Here's your must-have info on caring for winter-vulnerable skin, a pre-ski workout, stay-supple stretches and night-time glamour for high-voltage looks.

# Stay well in winter

Protecting your health and wellbeing means taking extra care during the cold weather season when the number of viruses circulating increases dramatically. Why this increase occurs, scientists do not yet know, but we can at least protect ourselves by watching out for resistance-lowering factors in our lifestyles and focusing our attention on keeping our immune systems working at peak efficiency.

Nutritional elements essential for a healthy immune system are zinc, calcium, magnesium, vitamins A, B complex, C, E and selenium. Vitamin A is vital, making cell walls stronger and so helping to protect against the invasion of viruses, advises nutrition consultant Jennifer Meek. She recommends 20,000 iu of vitamin A daily, Buy the beta-carotene form from health food shops and chemists throughout the winter. Vitamin C, with calcium and magnesium, increases the body's production of interferon, an infection fighter. Take 1 g or more each day during the cold months.

The immune army can be severely weakened by poor diet. Alcohol, cigarettes, saturated fat, refined carbohydrates and sugar should all be avoided. Jennifer Meek points to fat particularly. 'Fat is absorbed into the lymph vessels, slowing the system.' It is the lymph system which provides two-way transportation of antibodies and toxic waste. Lymph fluid is circulated by muscle activity – making movement and exercise especially important at this time of the year. Drink lots of water to flush away toxins created when cells are under viral attack.

The immune system is also adversely affected by stress. Research has shown that we often fall prey to colds when we suffer an upset such as changing jobs, moving home or divorce. When under stress, the body produces corticosteroids, which are very powerful immuno-suppressants. They also burn up zinc and B vitamins, especially B6 which is imperative for optimum immune function.

## COLD ACTION PLAN
*If you have the slightest sign of a cold starting – red, watery eyes or a runny nose – or if you have been in contact with someone who has a cold, use this action plan to shorten a cold's lifespan and lessen the severity of the symptoms.*

*✳ There is evidence to suggest that zinc is effective. Suck zinc gluconate tablets.*

*✳ Many studies have demonstrated vitamin C's cold-fighting potential. However, just as many more have shown unclear results. Nutritionists believe the key to success is in the dosage – an average of 2,000 mg (two 1 g tablets) is recommended every 3 hours. Some people need less, some more. If you get diarrhoea or stomach pain you will need less.*

# WINTER ZEST

*Drink plenty of liquids. Researchers at Harvard Medical School, in their book* Your Good Health *(edited by Bennett, Goldfinger and Johnson) comment, 'It's fair to say that a modest increase of vitamin C taken during a cold often makes people feel better, even when they don't know they are taking it. The effect is enhanced if subjects know or guess they are taking the vitamin. Psychology also plays a part in the severity of colds. One study showed that introverts have more severe cold symptoms than extroverts.*

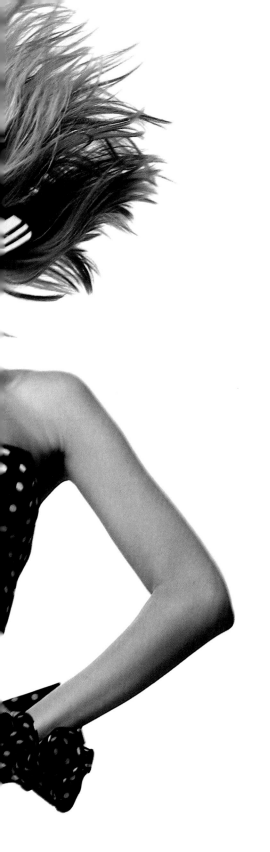

* *Although being in a stuffy environment doesn't help, keeping warm does. The immune system works better when hot.*

* **Homeopathic remedies:**
*Needs will depend on the symptoms and the time of year you catch the cold. Check with a homeopathic doctor or chemist. When self-treating with over-the-counter remedies, advises homeopath Dr Andrew Lockie, start the remedy the minute the symptoms appear but check with a doctor if your fever lasts over 48 hours or you have a temperature higher than 38.5°C (101°F).*

* **Aromatherapy:** *Many essential oils are anti-viral and anti-bacterial. Look for ready-mixed natural health remedies containing essential oils. Or place a few drops of an oil in a water spray and spritz your home and office, tissues and pillows. Check the aromatherapy guide on pages 126–129.*

* **Herbal help:** *Lime flower, elderflower, lemon balm, sage and rosemary are some of the herbs that help ease cold symptoms. Drink them as infusions or as ready-prepared herbal teas.*

# **g**et fit for skiing

If you're tired and underfit you're more likely to come a cropper. Start training 6–8 weeks before you go with a pre-ski routine at home or body conditioning classes which include resistance-training to build muscle, plus aerobics classes or activities that increase your cardio-vascular fitness (stamina). Cycling is an excellent activity to include in your exercise programme, as is swimming, but both should be done regularly.

On the slopes, check your muscles are warm and do stretching exercises before you race off.

## YOUR PRE-SKI WORKOUT

**W**arm up your muscles before you begin. Repeat each exercise 8 times.

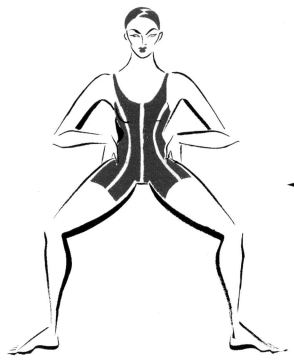

1. THIGHS AND CALVES: Stand with legs shoulder-width apart, slowly bend and straighten knees, lowering buttocks 15 cm (6 inches). Do this slowly being careful to keep back flat and in line with hips.

Note: Don't allow knees to turn in – keep them over feet.

◀ 2. FULL SQUATS (also good for thighs and calves): Stand with legs shoulder-width apart, lower buttocks until they are in line with knees and hold the position for 8 seconds.
**Note:** Don't let buttocks go lower than the knees and don't allow knees to roll in.

3. CALF EXERCISES: Stand with arms straight out in front, legs straight, feet straight and together. Rise up on toes. Hold the position for 8 seconds and then lower. Repeat 8 times. Then, with feet flat on floor, bend forward at the knees 8 times.

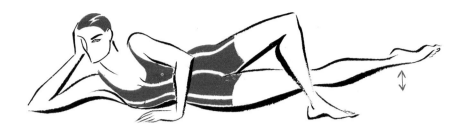

4. **INNER THIGH:** Lie on one side, propped up on elbow, bottom leg straight, top leg bent over thigh of bottom leg with whole foot in contact with the floor. Hold stomach in and lift bottom leg up and down with control 8 times slowly. Then make 16 small, quicker repetitions at the top of the movement. Repeat on other side.

5. **SKI-TURN:** Stand with arms straight out at sides, heels on the edge of a 7.5 cm (3-inch) thick mat. Bend knees as in skiing position. Swivel feet and knees from side to side.

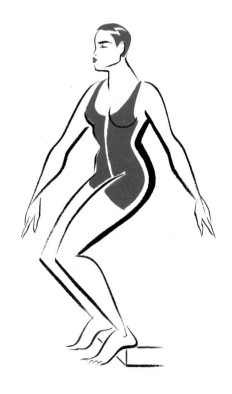

6. **ARMS (TRICEPS):** Sit with knees bent, feet flat on floor. Place hands behind you, palms on floor, fingers pointing forwards. Lift bottom off floor. Holding body still, bend arms and straighten. Feel weight of body in backs of arms (triceps).
**Note:** Don't lift shoulders or allow your body to make the movement.

WINTER *ZEST*

7. ARMS (BICEPS): Standing with knees bent and pelvis tucked under, hold a 900 g (2 lb) bag of sugar, or anything manageable of similar weight, in each hand. Keep elbows tucked into waist and bring both hands in towards shoulders. Lower but do not fully straighten arms. Repeat 10 times slowly and smoothly and 20 times more quickly in the middle of the range of movement.

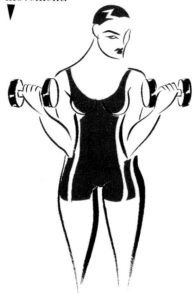

*Headed for the slopes? You're also headed for one of the toughest workouts you can take on – skiing. Skiing demands stamina – masses of it – suppleness, agility, co-ordination, strength in the legs, thighs and the upper body.*

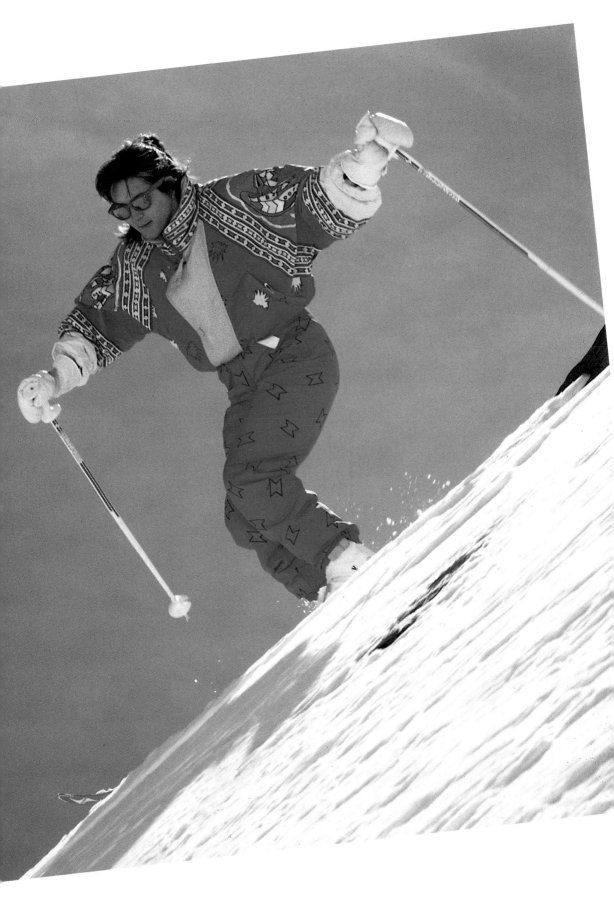

# **m**assage

Masseur and natural beauty expert Clare Maxwell-Hudson suggests this simple neck and shoulder massage which can be done through a partner's or friend's clothes, while they are watching the television, or listening to some favourite relaxing music. In just a few minutes, you can relieve tense muscles and calm feelings of anxiety. You should not massage, however, if the person is feeling unwell, or has a medical condition. The movements, when massaging, should not be painful and should avoid the spine.

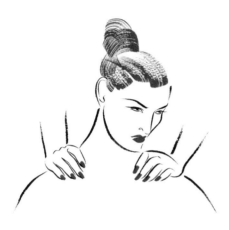

1. With your partner sitting in a chair, stand behind and place your hands on the tops of their shoulders. Press down, using your body weight to apply pressure, and then relax. Repeat several times. ▲

3. With both hands together on the ▶ right hand side of the neck, knead the shoulders and arms by squeezing first one hand and then the other as though kneading dough, moving across the tops of the shoulders and down the upper arms, and then back again. Knead on the other side. Repeat 2 more times.
Return to stroking – in massage, you always alternate between a firm, working movement and a soothing, calming movement. Repeat 6 times or more.

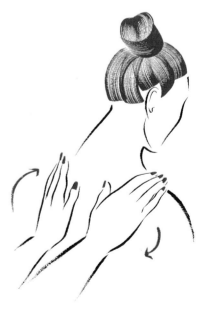

2. Firmly stroke the shoulders and upper back, circling the right hand clockwise, the left hand anti-clockwise. Repeat 6 times. ▶

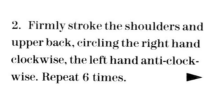

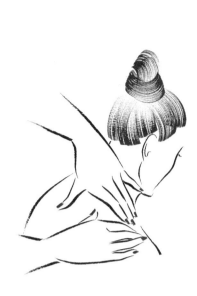

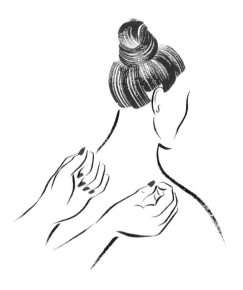

5.  Next, a stimulating pummelling movement. With the fleshy parts of lightly closed fists (the sides of the hands by the little fingers) – and remembering not to touch the spine – pummel the shoulders and back with both hands together, flicking the hands up and away.
Switch to gentle kneading and stroking.

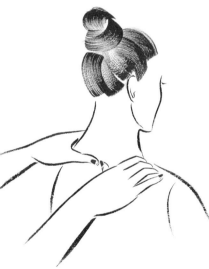

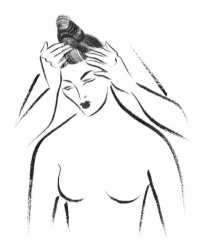

4.  Rest your hands on top of your partner's shoulders, thumbs on either side of the spine. Using deep, rotating movements, circle on the spot. Release the pressure and move up about 2.5 cm (1 inch), working up towards the neck.
To massage the neck, place one hand on the forehead to support the head and use the thumb and first fingers of the other hand to circle on either side of the spine. Stroke the area again. ▲

6.  Place both hands very lightly on the forehead and, barely touching the skin, gently stroke down the neck, across the shoulders and down the arms. Repeat several times and finish by resting the hands lightly on the tops of the shoulders.

# breakfast boosters

**D**oes every working day kick off (badly) with the 'no-time-for breakfast' a.m. rush? You can look forward to breakfast – and save time – with these tastebud treats.

Make your breakfast a combination of protein and complex carbohydrates to put your mind on full alert and fuel your energy system.

✳ Porridge is a wonderful winter warmer: add a pinch of sea salt and brown sugar, a handful of raisins to rolled oats (or oatmeal) and water,

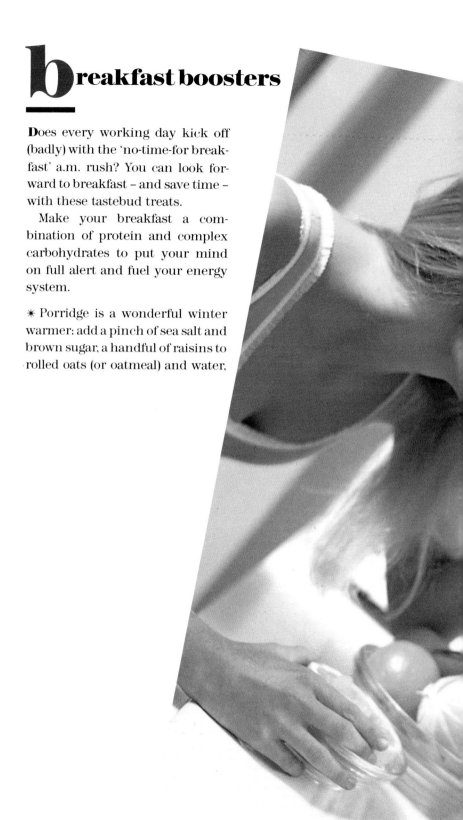

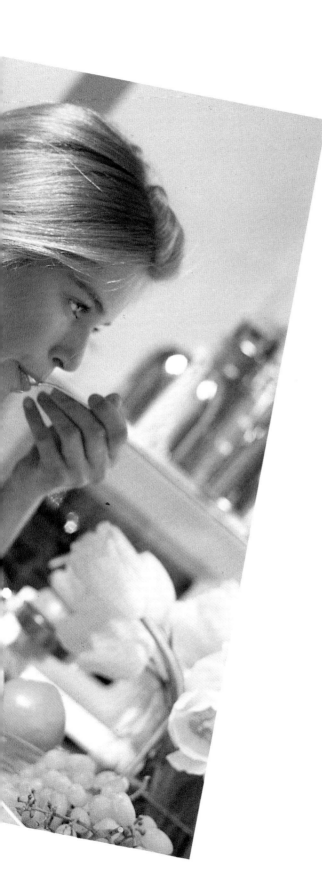

simmer (while you shower/dress) and serve with skimmed or semi-skimmed milk.

✳ Top cereals and porridge with chopped hazelnuts and seeds. Prepare mixes the night before and store in the refrigerator in a sealed bag or container.

✳ Dried fruit compote is a classic, delicious addition to cereal and yogurt and a good source of vitamins and fibre. Fill 2 cups, or mugs, with a mixture of dried prunes, peaches, apricots, figs, apples and raisins and place in a saucepan with the same amount of water. Add a stick of cinnamon and 2 slices of orange and 2 of lemon, unpeeled but scrubbed. Cover the saucepan, bring to the boil then remove from the heat. Serve chilled or warmed.

✳ Soak muesli and/or dried fruit overnight in apple juice for natural sweetness.

✳ Wholegrain bread is a good source of complex carbohydrates, plus B vitamins and fibre. This includes muffins and waffles! Skip the butter and enjoy a little sugar-free fruit spread.

✳ Low-fat yogurt provides protein and calcium. Add fresh fruit for a high-C source of energy, plus vitamin A.

✳ If you like to start the day with tea and coffee, but not the side-effects and short-term energy spurts of caffeine, look for water-processed decaffeinated coffee and teas. (Some decaff teas are undrinkable, others are delicious – so shop around.) **147**

# energy food

Perfect to keep to hand for an energy-boosting snack, and to add flavour and interest to breakfast cereals and salads, nuts and seeds are full of protein, essential vitamins and minerals.

*Nuts contain high levels of carbohydrate, fats and oils – particularly coconuts, Brazil and macadamia nuts – and shouldn't be turned into a feast! However (with the exception of coconut and pine nuts) they do contain linoleic acid which is believed to counteract the build-up of cholesterol from saturated fats and oils. Eat nuts in limited amounts, unless you're using them as a meat substitute.*

Seeds are a food source that will help you on the road to high-level health. They're high in beneficial polyunsaturated oils which help to enhance your complexion, fight heart disease and reduce inflammation. Look for whole, unchipped seeds when buying. Grind linseeds and sesame seeds in a coffee grinder to make them more digestible (unground sesame seeds are passed through your body whole). Grind enough for up to 3 days and refrigerate them in a clean, sealed jam jar.

*Check that the nuts you buy don't have any additives. Commercially packaged nuts often contain preservatives, and may be coated in saturated fats and salt.*

Don't hoard seeds and nuts for too long or they will go rancid. Unshelled nuts will keep for up to 6 months. Seeds and shelled nuts should be kept in a cool, dry, dark place in airtight containers. Chopped and ground nuts will go stale quickly and should be eaten within a few weeks. Roasting nuts will boost their flavour but reduce their nutritional value. Don't fry or roast seeds as the oils produce 'free radicals' (highly reactive molecules believed to be major factors in the ageing process).

## NUTS AND SEEDS: NUTRITIONAL STORE-HOUSES OF VITAMINS AND MINERALS

### Nuts

ALMONDS: Vitamin B2 (excellent), vitamin E, calcium (excellent), fibre, folic acid, iron, potassium.

BRAZIL NUTS: Vitamin B1, calcium, magnesium, potassium, zinc.

CASHEW NUTS: Vitamin A, folic acid, iron.

HAZELNUTS: Vitamin B6, vitamin E (excellent), fibre.

MACADAMIA NUTS: Not as nutritious as most other nuts; some vitamin B1, B2 and B3, calcium.

WALNUTS: Vitamin B6, folic acid, potassium.

### Seeds

PUMPKIN SEEDS: Vitamin A, iron.

SESAME SEEDS: Vitamin B3 (niacin), calcium, fibre, magnesium, zinc.

SUNFLOWER SEEDS: Vitamin A, vitamin B1, B3, B6, potassium, zinc.

## HEALTH CHECK: THE SOBER FACTS

You can't drink like a man. Women in general metabolize alcohol faster than men; a woman's blood alcohol level will rise higher for the same amount of alcohol as a man of the same weight; and women are more likely to experience memory loss and will perform worse in memory tests after drinking alcohol.

While in small quantities alcohol is relaxing and in studies has shown a preventive effect against coronary heart disease, heavy drinking is a health-breaker. For example – and these are just some of alcohol's side-kicks – women (who drink excessively) are also more at risk from cirrhosis of the liver. Alcohol has been linked to ovarian and breast cancer.

Check these guidelines to cut the health risks of drinking:

✳ Avoid alcohol just before a period, when you will be more vulnerable to its effects.

✳ Examine drinking habits at least once a year. While a drink may help to relieve stress, you should investigate the many other stress-beating solutions available. Whisk up non-alcoholic cocktails at home, and investigate low-alcohol and non-alcohol drinks when you are out.

✳ Hot weather enhances the brain's sensitivity to alcohol, increasing the chances of intoxication from even small amounts.

✳ Dilute the alcohol by drinking plenty of water at the same time.

✳ Take vitamin B complex – it supports the liver.

# Winterproof your skin

Whether head-first down the slopes, running along the beach, cycling in the park, hiking in the hills, or just walking around town – it's exhilarating to be out in the cold air, but wind, sun and low humidity are all hazards to skin condition that can mean dehydration (leading to fine lines and wrinkles), chapping and burning.

Moisture in the air drops as the temperature goes down and you will fare no better indoors where the heating leaves your skin tight and dry. And it's not only the elements that conspire against you. Your body actually produces less oil during cooler weather. Here's how to take extra care and beat the winter chill:

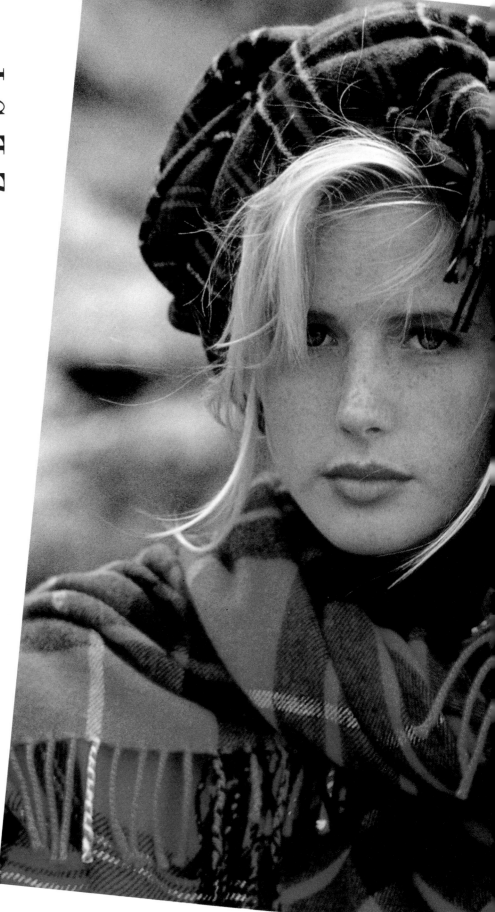

WINTER ZEST

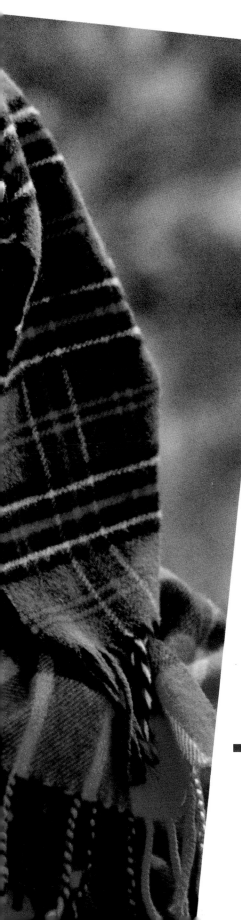

✳ Switch to a gentle facial cleanser. Read about the age-proofing movements you need to use for wipe-off lotions (page 156). Avoid shower gel – its high detergent content and direct application to the body can be overly harsh on winter skin. Likewise soaps: most are not PH balanced and over-strip the skin. Go for a cleansing bar instead.

✳ Check your skin isn't damp before going outside – it could chap in the wind.

✳ Change to a richer moisturizer – a cream rather than a lotion.

✳ As your skin reacts to the harsher conditions you may also need a night cream to help restore moisture lost during the day.

✳ If you're prone to broken capillaries and high colour avoid extremes of temperature – no dashing in from freezing temperatures to roast in front of the fire. Allow your skin to acclimatize first. Ideally, bring back circulation slowly by gently splashing the face with tepid, then warm, water.

✳ Use a humidifier, or place a pan of water on top of a radiator in your home and office to add moisture to the atmosphere.

*Anything that is absorbed into the skin too quickly is probably not sufficient.*

✴ Avoid peel-off masks. Instead, use a hydrating mask frequently to give your skin a blast of moisture.

✴ Those with oily skin tend to think they don't need to put anything on it. But moisture is still drawn away from the surface, resulting in skin that is dry and flaky on top but oily underneath. Cleanse regularly and *gently* exfoliate to remove dry surface skin. Choose protective gels or ampoules if your skin is prone to breakouts.

✴ Very dry skins should follow face cream with a foundation containing a moisturizer.

✴ Remember that hands take extra punishment during the winter. Smooth in a rich hand cream. This forms a layer over the skin to lock moisture in and prevent chapping and soreness.

## SKIN CARE FOR WINTER SPORTS

**D**ouble up on moisturizer, eye cream and lip balm before going out. Skin care specialist Lia Schorr recommends applying a layer of each, waiting 5 minutes and then re-applying. Keep the layers thin if you'll be sweating – running, cross-country skiing; thicker if you'll be hitting wind resistance – downhill skiing, skating, cycling – when the effect of cold air on the skin is much more drying.

*Use a sunscreen in place of your moisturizer and re-apply several times during the day. Use a skin protector even on a cloudy day – UV rays still penetrate and are far stronger at high altitudes. Use a 'block' on lips and nose as these will be extra-vulnerable. Opaque zinc oxide screens are really effective. Take lip protection over the sensitive edge of lips too. Sunscreens developed for skiing tend to have more occlusive, oilier formulations to seal in moisture and help beat the wind chill factor – if the water content of a product is too high it may freeze on the skin. Invest in products designed for this purpose – your summer sun-*

## CARED-FOR LIPS

Sensitive and vulnerable, lip tissue is almost defenceless. Unlike the rest of your skin, it contains no melanin to protect against UV rays, no sebaceous glands to provide moisture and prevent cracking and no sweat glands for temperature regulation. Moisture-loss occurs faster because the outer layer of skin is much thinner. The result: lip surfaces can become dehydrated, leading to creased, cracking and peeling skin. In addition, wrinkles develop around the mouth with deep vertical grooves extending into the lip line.

✴ Strengthen and protect your lips with creams and balms formulated to maintain the moisture balance.

✴ Waxy balms provide the most effective barrier against moisture loss, essential when you're skiing and useful if you frequently lick or chew your lips or if you have a cold.

✴ If your lips do become chapped don't be tempted to peel or pull at the skin – you'll damage the underlying structure of the lips and leave them open to infection. Choose a soothing or repairing product which may contain active ingredients to stimulate the blood circulation and encourage faster healing.

✴ Creating a smooth surface for lipstick is tricky on creased or rough, chapped lips. Make-up artist Kim Jacob applies a little vaseline before foundation, then blots off greasiness with a tissue before applying any lipstick. Lip fixes and primers work in the same way, filling in creases, and also provide fixing agents to give your lipstick staying power.

*screens will be lighter, and have less oil, although if your skin is prone to acne, you should use a ski screen on trouble-free zones and normal sunblock elsewhere.*

**W**ear high-quality goggles or sunglasses to protect skin around eyes.

*Any redness or soreness should be treated gently. Use a cream cleanser, mild toner and moisturize with a richer cream than usual. Don't peel off chapped skin on the face or lips. You can gently exfoliate dry skin on the face when redness has gone, treating the skin to moisturizer afterwards.*

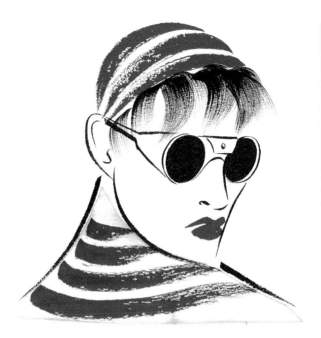

# **g**reat skin at your fingertips

**C**heck out the terrific benefits of a refreshing facial that's fast and easy to do at home. It gives an instant boost to a tired or sallow complexion, improves the skin's texture, and reduces any tendency to redness or broken capillaries. Your skin will be less prone to breakouts or blocked pores. And even your eyes will look brighter once puffiness is smoothed away.

The movements shown overleaf will stimulate the circulation of lymph – the fluid that carries away toxins. Unlike blood, the lymphatic system has no pumping station but is activated by muscle movement. In your face, with its complex bone structure, these muscles can easily become congested. Use this lymphatic drainage massage as an important part of your skin fitness routine 2 or 3 times a week (or more if you have problem skin). Eve Lom, the skin specialist who developed it, suggests doing it as you cleanse in the evening, as the movements are gentle and soothing. Use the pads of your fingers and close your eyes so that you can relax and sense the pressure.

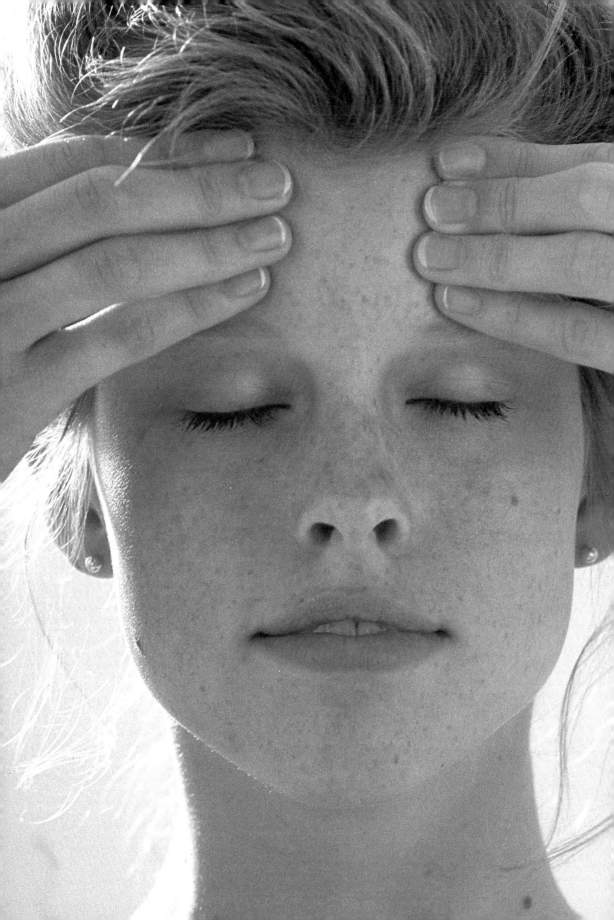

# *Healthy, glowing skin is a few short steps away with this fabulous facial.*

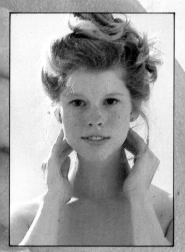
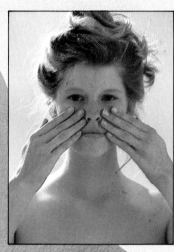
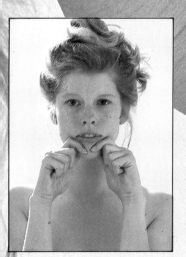
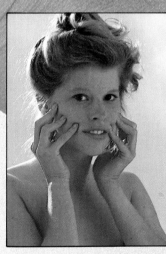

1. Smooth a slippery cleanser over the face and neck or apply a little essential oil or massage cream so that fingertips glide over, and don't pull, the skin. Beginning behind the ears to clear the lymphatic channels for the rest of the face, apply deep pressure and circle down to the collar-bone.

2. Place fingers in centre of forehead, from browbone to hairline. The key movement is: press firmly for a count of 3, then release. Move fingers apart by 12 mm (½ inch), press, hold and release again. Repeat finishing at temples.

3. Starting under the eyes, press down along the bridge of the nose to the corners of the mouth. Repeat the movement several times around the mouth.

4. With thumbs under chin and index fingers at centre, press-release along the jawbone, finishing under the ears.

5. Place the fingers, spread like a fan, under the cheekbones and press-release down to jawline. Place the palms of the hands flat against the neck, fingers behind ears and circle firmly 5 times.

To complete the facial, use hot and cold compresses to help the removal of toxins. Hold a cloth soaked in hot water to the face (not so hot that it's uncomfortable, though). Gently remove the cleanser, oil or massage cream and repeat twice more. Follow with a cold water compress (again don't go for extreme cold).

# the skin refresher course

Winter skin needs extra-gentle cleansing. Right now, one thing's for sure – soap and water are out. They're too harsh, too drying for weather-buffeted skin. Switch to a wash-off or wipe-off cleanser and learn to use the lightest possible touch and kindest movements (see below). Milky or cream cleansers are winners when it comes to removing make-up. And chances are you're wearing more make-up at this time of the year (a) to protect against the elements and seal in moisture and (b) to liven up a pallid complexion.

## CLEANSING: THE HEALTHY SKIN ROUTINE

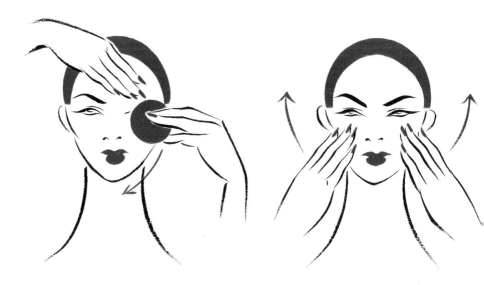

1. Remove eye make-up. Eyes need special care because the skin in this area is very delicate and oil which gets into the eye could lead to irritation and puffiness, so use a water-based eye make-up remover. Soak 2 cotton wool pads in the lotion. Using one pad for each eye (to avoid spreading any infection), hold it to the lashes for a few seconds to dissolve the make-up, then stroke in *towards* the nose and down from the brow – moving up and out pulls the skin in the wrong direction.

2. Warm the cleanser in your hands first: if it goes on cold, your pores will 'close up', making removal of dirt more difficult. Smooth it over your face with the whole hand starting at the neck and working in upward and outward movements. Then put your thumbs under your chin and work little circles around your nose and chin to dislodge trapped dirt. Remove by blotting and wiping gently with a soft tissue.

## THE SKIN BOOSTER

Use an exfoliator once or twice a week to remove dead skin cells – it will help your complexion to look fresher, refining the texture, and help moisturizer to penetrate, especially if your skin is dry and flaky. Use the same upward and outward movements as for cleansing, circling lightly and resting your thumbs under your chin when you focus on the nose and chin. Some exfoliating creams and cleansing pads are too tough.

### Take care that you:

* *Always use the gentlest product you can find*

* *Don't slough acned skin or skin prone to breakout without your doctor's advice*

* *Don't rub or scrub. The skin should not change colour*

* *Don't use exfoliators on the lips or in the eye areas.*

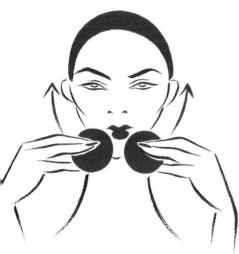

3. Use an efficient toner to remove last traces of grime and cleanser, then you shouldn't need to use soap or rinsable cleanser after removing make-up. Sweep on gently with upward and outward movements, avoiding the eye area. Blot skin dry with a tissue.

**Note:** Not all skin experts advocate exfoliation for the face. Some believe that massage is the key to exercising the skin. If your skin is delicate and sensitive or prone to spots, try a deep-cleansing mask instead on needy areas or use the facial massage on pages 154–155.

# *ZEST*

# **S**tretch your flexibility

**S**tretching muscles improves flexibility, suppleness, and joint mobility, helps you to maintain correct posture and to prevent muscle tears and over-use injuries, but it should be done carefully. In fact, it is believed that muscles do not actually stretch, they just relax more fully.

Try to hold stretches for at least 30 seconds and *don't bounce*. Stretch to the point of tightness, not pain. Beware of hyperextending. Constant over-stretching of your muscles will affect the ligaments. Joint injuries and other problems can be caused where the joint is no longer stabilized. Stretch must always be balanced by strength. Never stand and bend over at the waist without first bending the knees – bending to touch the floor with the knees locked and back rounded is known as 'the slipped disc position'.

Avoid stretches such as 'the plough' (where you lie on your back and bring your hips and feet over the head) unless you are really advanced and have done them with a properly trained instructor.

*Stretching is enjoyable – and an important part of being fit and healthy.*

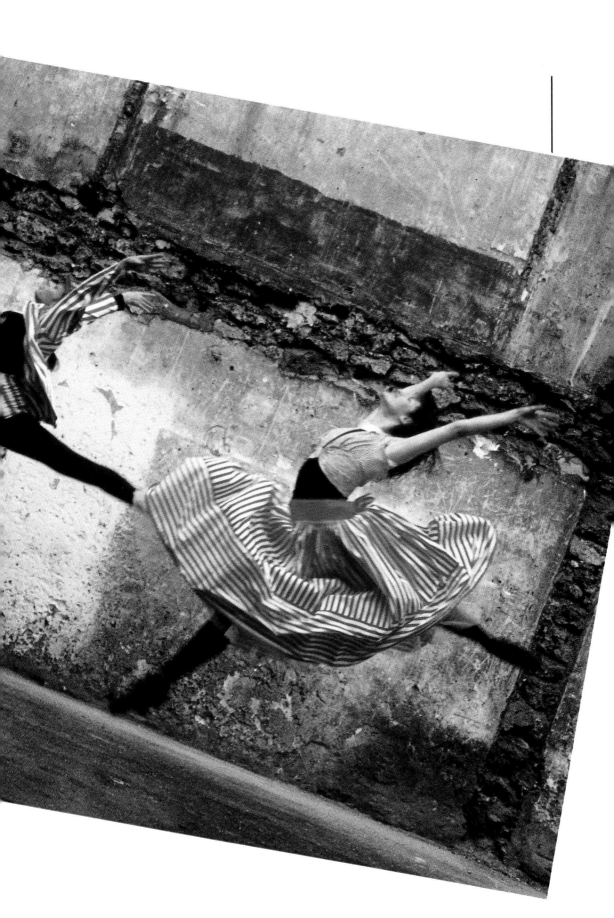

## DANCERS' STRETCHES

Follow in the footsteps of classical and contemporary dancers: Increase your energy levels, improve flexibility and strengthen your muscles with this simple stretching sequence you can use every day.

Before you begin, make sure that your body is really warm. Start with an energizing stretch. Breathe in deeply through your nose, raising your arms and feeling your chest expand. Breathe out through your lips as you lower arms. Perform each movement for a slow count of 4 and repeat each one 4 times.

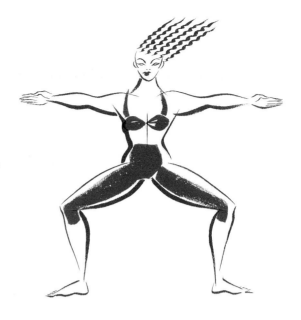

1.  Pliés: Every dancer's limber for the inner thigh, groin and hips. Stand with legs 75 cm (2½ ft) apart, thighs turned outwards from the hips so that when you bend your knee it falls over your foot and does not roll inwards; arms at sides. Breathe in and raise arms to shoulder level (keeping shoulders down). Breathe out and bend knees slowly, keeping back straight. Breathe in slowly, straightening legs. ▲

2.  Hip release and spiral stretch: ▶ Bring your feet in together and raise your arms to shoulder level to help your balance. Draw your right foot up your left leg towards your knee, keeping the thigh turned outwards (breathing in for 4 counts). Hold position for a count of 4, breathing out. Now breathe in and move knee across body. At the same time, place left arm over leg, so that you can press the thigh into your body and gently twist around to the right, creating a spiral effect. Hold position for a count of 4, breathing out. Breathe in and turn the leg out again. Breathe out and take your leg and arms down. Repeat on other leg.

**Note:** To help you balance, keep your stomach muscles pulled in. Pull up the front thigh muscles of the leg you're standing on.

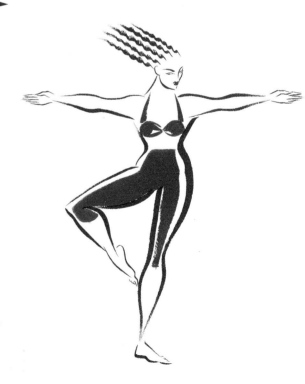

3. Calf stretch: Put right leg directly behind you with foot facing forwards, heel down on ground. Breathe out as you take your weight forwards, bending front leg and hold (make sure your knee points over your foot to keep the joint stable and does not turn in), feeling the stretch in calf of back leg. Breathe in as you slowly come up and go into stretch again. Work both sides. As your calf muscle begins to release gradually bend forwards. ▼

4. Hamstring stretch: You should feel this stretch in the back of the legs. Keep feet parallel and breathe out as you bend forwards from the hips **without rounding your back**. Aim to create a straight line from base of spine to top of head. Repeat with other leg. ▼

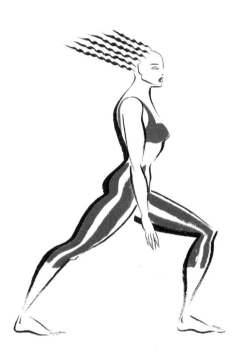

5. Side stretch: Standing with right ► leg in front of left (as in calf stretch), stretch left arm forwards, right arm back, breathing in. Breathe out and gently twist body towards right as you stretch up with left arm. Feel stretch up left side of body. Breathe in, bringing arms down and repeat 3 more times. Put left leg in front and repeat, stretching away with right arm.

# **m**ake-up fast

1. Cleanse your face and apply a moisturizer where you need it, ideally one that contains ultra-violet screens. Tinted moisturizer gives a quick glow if you don't need foundation. Give the moisturizer a couple of minutes on your skin before applying foundation – you can clean your teeth and brush your hair while you're waiting.

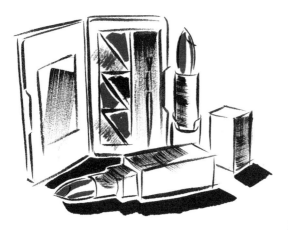

*Make-up applied with professional polish can look great throughout the working day. Adapt your make-up routine to the busiest a.m. schedule with these beat-the-clock tips.*

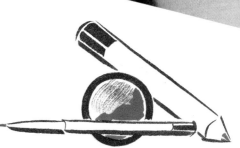

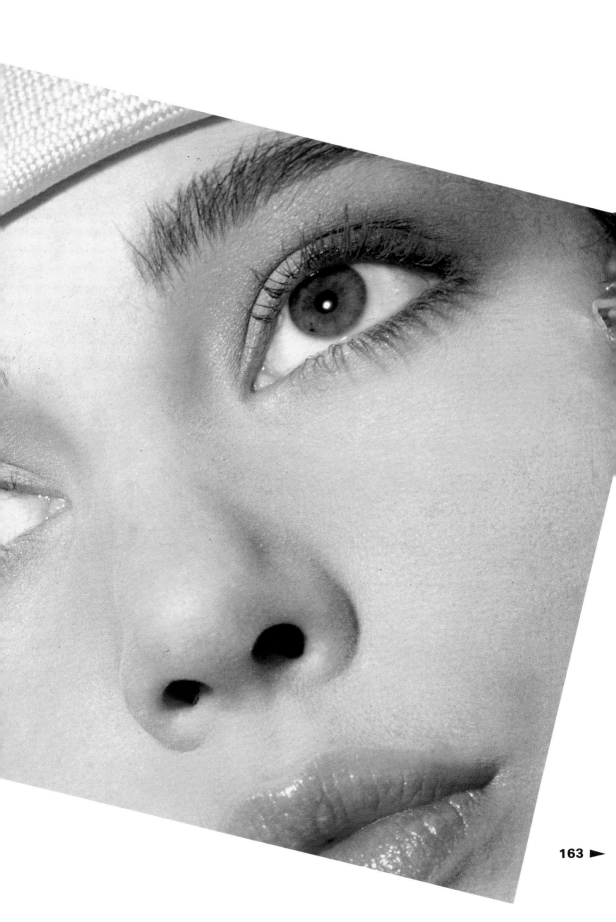

Make-up fast continued

2. Apply foundation, if you wear it, using downward and outward strokes. Start in the centre, blending out towards, but not into, the hairline, and fade out as you reach under the jawline (don't take foundation down on to the neck). A sheer finish looks contemporary and fresh for day – don't try to cover skin texture, just even out your skin tone.

3. Cover any blemishes or dark rings with concealer using a flat brush.

4. Press on a powder with a translucent finish, or one that gives a warm, beige glow. Fluff off any excess with a big brush. If you don't wear foundation, still use powder to avoid looking un-made-up and to help keep your blusher and eye colours looking good longer.

5. Follow with honey, coral or pink blusher on cheeks and use it to double up as eyeshadow if you like. Cream or gel blusher looks most natural. Powder blusher is longer-lasting in warm weather.

*Light, muted colours stand up to fast application. Dark, dramatic shades require time and precision.*

6. Define brows, if necessary, with a pencil. Brush them upwards to enlarge your eyes – this can work wonders if you don't have time for mascara (and if you don't have bushy eyebrows).

7. Eyeliner gives instant emphasis – draw along your top lid close to lashes. If using a pencil eyeliner, smudge lightly with a cotton bud or eyeshadow applicator.

8. Keep eye colour understated – use matte browns, peach or pink shades and blend well. The new waterproof, crease-resistant pencils and creams are great for day-long city wear.

9. Apply a quick coat of mascara – just to top lashes if you're tight on time. It will also prevent smudging underneath the eye which can make eyes look tired. Don't wear water-proof mascara every day – it's drying and takes a lot of removing.

10. *To finish:* no time for lipliner! Apply lipstick with a clean square eyeshadow brush, recommends make-up artist Amanda Jackson-Sytner – the larger size means colour goes on faster. Or use fingers to apply just enough colour to stain lips. Retouch during the day.

## QUICK DAY-TO-NIGHT TURNAROUNDS

✳ Keep a gold or bronze eyeshadow and a sexy red or shimmery lipstick and matching lipliner in your desk drawer.

✳ Changing lip colour is faster and just as effective as changing your eye colour.

## NIGHT TIME SPARKLE

**G**o all out for glamour! Set temperatures soaring with smouldering eyes, the most luminous skin and the hottest lips. Here's how to gleam for evening, from start to finish.

**S**witch on some music and apply a spritz of perfume to put you in a party mood. Check that your face is brightly and evenly lit with artificial light.

**F**or sure-fire success don't experiment the same evening that you're due out!

**A**pply moisturizer 5–10 minutes before your foundation. If your skin is dry and flaky, the base will go patchy.

**C**reate a perfect palette: consider using a complexion primer if your skin needs extra help – they are white, designed to reflect the light and impart a luminous glow. Or use a colour corrector – green to tone down redness, just in the areas you need it, lilac to boost a sallow complexion.

**A**pply foundation to the back of your hand, and then dot on to nose, forehead, chin and cheeks. Damp a make-up sponge, squeeze out in a towel or tissue. Some make-up artists prefer a dry sponge – experiment to find which works best with your foundation formulation. Blend in a downwards direction, fading out towards the hairline and under jawline. Be very sparing under the eyes – too much can set in the lines.

**A**pply concealer with a lip brush to prevent caking.

*The key to applying and blending matte and semi-matte eyeshadows super-successfully: use a 'primer' of translucent loose powder or off-white matte eyeshadow first.*

**P**ress powder in with a compact puff and stroke lightly in every direction to cover your face completely. Use a big brush, and downward and outward strokes to remove any excess.

**N**ow warm up your base with a hint of blusher. Smile and apply blusher from the centre of your cheeks out to your temples (but not into the hairline). Use a good-sized brush – many of the brushes in blusher compacts are too small for a soft, natural finish.

**D**efine brows to frame your eyes with a little mascara or eyebrow make-up. Or simply brush up lightly.

**A**pply a liberal dusting of translucent powder under the eye before you use eyeshadow. Any loose pigment can then be swept off afterwards with a large soft brush.

**O**ff-white eyeshadow applied from lid to brow makes a good base and will help prevent eye make-up creasing. Then, define eyes with a smoky toned pencil or kohl line.

*ZEST*

Make-up fast continued

*Apply the most dramatic colour next. Check your applicator isn't overloaded with eyeshadow by tapping it gently over a tissue before applying. Glittery, gleaming loose shadows can be especially tricky to apply. Damp the make-up applicator lightly to control the colour and increase its staying power.*

*You can use translucent powder to create a smooth, blended effect on the eyes, advises visagiste Ray Allington. Just add a little powder to the tip of your brush to make blending one colour into another easier.*

*Pull back from the mirror and check the effect as you go. Use a magnifying mirror too if you can.*

*Using a light colour under the eye will brighten tired-looking eyes. But don't use it if your eyes are prominent – instead, use a dark colour inside the lid for a sultry, glamorous style.*

*Take eye colour up into brows to increase the dramatic effect.*

*Eyelash curlers are indispensable. Get as close to the lashline as possible. Now apply 2 coats of mascara, letting the first coat dry before sweeping on the second. Coloured mascara looks vibrant and exciting for evening.*

*Balance your look: Set bright, colourful eyes against pale cheeks and softly shaded lips. Or make lips lively and exciting and use smoky shadow or liner on the eyes.*

*Outline lips with matching or paler toned lipliner, apply a first coat of lipstick, then separate a tissue and blot with one ply. Brush a little translucent powder over lips, re-apply lipstick and blot again. If you find bright lip colour difficult to apply, fill in corners with a lip pencil instead of using a brush or lipstick.*

*Using shimmering rose pink blusher if you are pale skinned, or copper if you are darker, on shoulders, in the cleavage and the hollows of your neck adds to the high wattage effect.*

*Don't forget nail varnish to make you feel really polished!*

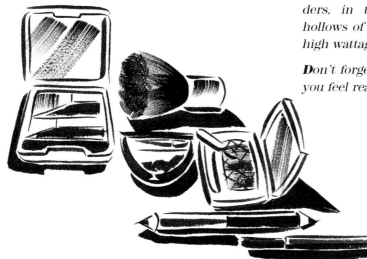

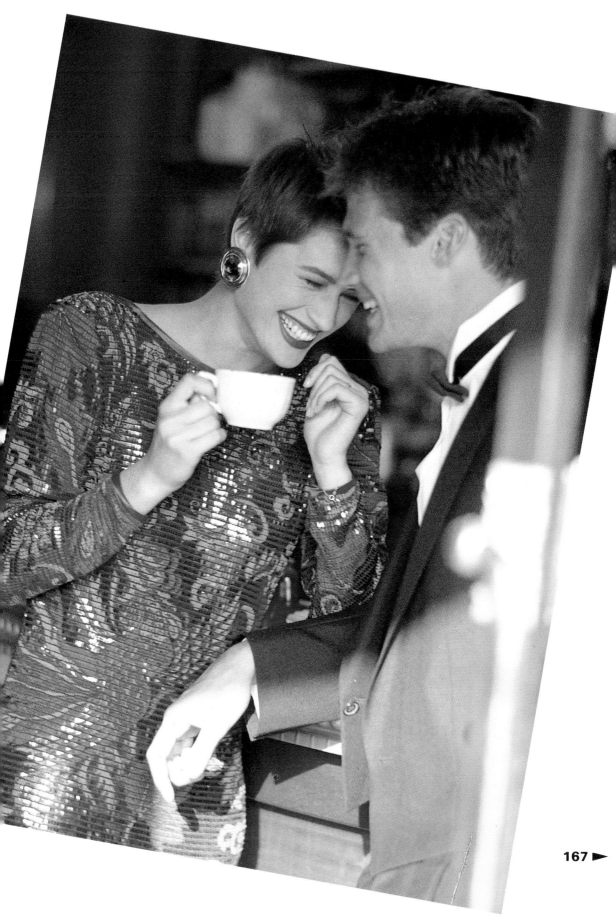

# **n**utrition

**WHAT IS A BALANCED DIET?**
Most people believe they already have a balanced diet. However, in a recent study, although almost everyone interviewed – 320 women – believed they followed a balanced diet, only one in 10 received even the minimum of nutrients to fulfil the UK's recommended daily allowances (RDAs).

The best way to achieve a balanced, healthy diet is to leave out the negatives – foods which are known to be damaging. These include coffee, salt, sugar and additives and preservatives. Concentrate on the positives – foods which are highest in nutrients: this means unprocessed foods. That doesn't just mean wholefoods, such as grains, nuts and seeds, it also means wholefoods that are not over-cooked. If you cook healthy brown rice for an hour, it ends up as very simple, non-nutritious carbohydrate. So it's not just a matter of what you buy, but what you do to it.

*Are we eating a balanced diet? Do we need to take vitamin supplements?* Patrick Holford of the Institute for Optimum Nutrition supplies the answers.

**ARE VITAMIN AND MINERAL SUPPLEMENTS NECESSARY?**
*Nutritionists often argue that vitamin and mineral supplements are not necessary, on the basis that the recommended daily allowances (RDAs) of these substances are provided in any reasonably normal diet. Nevertheless, there are arguments in favour of supplementing: The current framework for vitamin RDAs, on which nutritionists base their claims, is to look at the smallest amount needed to prevent an obvious deficiency, rather than provide optimum health. In addition, British RDAs have not been updated for over 30 years; those established in other countries such as the USA are the result of new research.*

✳ *Growing and storing conditions, and the length of time food is kept can all affect vitamin levels – there is evidence to suggest that fruit and vegetables kept for some time in supermarkets, for example, suffer loss of vitamin content. Replace fresh vegetables and fruit frequently with new stocks and keep them in a cool dark place. Environmental factors may also play a part: in England diets are very low in zinc, selenium, chromium and manganese because the levels in the soil are too low for optimum health. This is because areas that were glaciated thousands of years ago were robbed of various minerals in the topsoil.*

Vitamin and mineral needs can fluctuate. Vitamin C requirements, for example, will vary according to pollution and stress levels (smoking will use up 20 mg per cigarette). We are all biochemically different and our vitamin and mineral needs will vary enormously from individual to individual.

✷ A hectic lifestyle can often foil our good intentions for healthy eating. How often do you rush home late and grab a pre-pack from the freezer or open a tin? When food is processed many of the vitamins and minerals are stripped away and not all are put back. As legislation stands, calcium, magnesium and iron are the only minerals which have to be replaced if they're refined out.

✷ Methods of food preparation – soaking, chopping and cooking – can deplete vitamin content. Levels fall even further if food is kept hot. The best way to retain vitamins and flavour is by steaming or pressure-cooking.

✷ Women have special vitamin needs. The menstrual cycle puts extra stress on the body each month; iron in particular is lost. The contraceptive pill affects the body's supplies of B6.

---

**Note:** Vitamin and mineral therapy – treating specific conditions with groups of nutrients – should only be undertaken with the advice of highly trained nutritionists. Never take large, or 'mega' doses of supplements without medical supervision.

*Aim to make up half of your diet from raw foods – fruits and vegetables, nuts and seeds, live yogurt, sprouted pulses. The other half should be cooked whole grains, low-fat cheese, eggs, fish and a little meat, mainly white.*

---

### CAN NUTRIENTS AFFECT OUR MOODS?

The first thing that is affected through a nutritional imbalance is your state of mind. Seventy per cent of the body's energy is used by the brain, so it's logical that this should always be the first place to register an imbalance. The Swedish research scientist in nutrition, Dr Carl Pfieffer, has found that 50% of schizophrenics have a zinc deficiency.

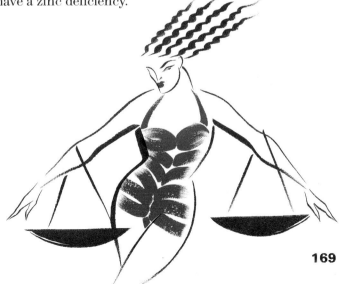

WINTER *ZEST*

## SUPPLEMENTS: SUGGESTED DAILY REQUIREMENTS

If you are considering taking supplements, check this list of average daily requirements and good food sources.

## Vitamins

VITAMIN A 7,500 iu: Carrots, root vegetables, sweet potatoes, spinach, cheese, milk, eggs, apricots, liver

VITAMIN B1 (Thiamin) 50 mg: Wholemeal bread, brown rice, pulses, yeast extract, cornflakes, meat – especially pork

VITAMIN B2 (Riboflavin) 50 mg: Liver, Cheddar cheese, milk, meat, cereals, wholemeal bread

VITAMIN B3 (Niacin) 50 mg: Chicken, lean meat, liver, green beans, pulses, cereals

VITAMIN B5 (Pantothenic acid) 50 mg: Meat, eggs, fish, molasses, brewer's yeast, chicken

VITAMIN B6 (Pyridoxine) 50 mg: Wheatgerm, bananas, turkey, yeast, eggs, wholegrain cereal

VITAMIN B12 5–10 mcg: Meat, eggs, milk, spirulina. Vegetarians are advised to take supplements

VITAMIN C 1 g: Blackcurrants, citrus fruits, green vegetables, green peppers

VITAMIN D 400 iu: Eggs, oily fish, margarine, fortified milk. (We also make vitamin D from sunlight)

VITAMIN E 100 iu: Many foods, including vegetable oils, milk, eggs, nuts, seeds

VITAMIN K: Green vegetables, turnips, cereals. (Also produced by bacteria in the intestines). Supplements not required

BIOTIN 50 mcg: Dairy produce. (Also produced by bacteria in the intestines)

FOLIC ACID 50 mcg: Green vegetables

BIOFLAVINOIDS 25 mg: Citrus fruits, green peppers

## Minerals

CALCIUM 500 mg: Milk (look for fortified milk if buying skimmed), cheese, green vegetables, broccoli, nuts, seeds, pulses

IRON 12 mg: Liver, kidneys, egg yolk, cane molasses, pulses

ZINC 15 mg: Meat, nuts, eggs, wholewheat, rye, oats, milk, carrots

MAGNESIUM 350 mg: Green vegetables, eggs, milk, bread, meat, peanuts

POTASSIUM 20 mg: All vegetables, bananas, dandelion coffee

IODINE 140 mcg: Fish and seafood, eggs, peanuts, cereals. Supplements not required

COPPER 2.5 mg: Most foods, especially oysters, kidneys, pulses, nuts. Supplements not required

SELENIUM 20 mcg: Seafood, beans, seeds, especially sesame seeds

CHROMIUM 20 mcg: Wholegrains, mushrooms, asparagus, pulses

MANGANESE 5 mg: Tropical fruits, pulses

# **b**oost your energy levels

## SYSTEM-SLOWERS

Fatigue is the leading health complaint of young women. Of a long list of possible causes, the following are common culprits:

✳ Wintry weather, centrally heated rooms and shorter days can leave you feeling sluggish and slow. Get out in the daylight every day – go for a walk with the dog, for a chat with a friend.

✳ Sleepless nights caused by stress and/or drinking caffeine or alcohol. Limit your caffeine intake (tea contains less than coffee) and don't drink it past mid-afternoon. Restrict your alcohol intake and don't drink before bedtime. Leave the hour before bed to wind down rather than trying to finish the work you didn't complete today!

✳ If you're feeling low, do some vigorous exercise – you'll stimulate mood-improving hormones and enhance your self-esteem.

✳ Your energy may dip during your menstrual cycle. Eat iron-rich foods such as spinach, eggs and lean red meat or take iron tablets, and ease up at work and on exercise when menstruating.

✳ We often *think* ourselves tired, says Donald Norfolk in his book *Farewell to Fatigue* (Michael Joseph). We come home after a tedious journey and expect to feel jaded. We could just as easily imagine ourselves fresh and lively.

✳ Fighting an infection taxes energy reserves. Medications, particularly antihistamines found in travel sickness tablets and allergy pills, antibiotics and anti-depressants can cause tiredness, as can the contraceptive pill.

✳ Dieting is frequently a cause of low energy. Don't use very low calorie diets.

## VITALITY BOOSTERS

**Take a walk!** *Researchers at California State University have found that a 10-minute walk is better at beating after-lunch lethargy than a break and a chocolate bar. Walkers reported that they felt tension levels were lower and their energy higher as much as 2 hours after breaking for the stroll. Sugar snackers had a short-term boost from their 'sugar fix' but an hour later felt as tired as before and even more tense.*

**Time to get strong:** *The weaker your body is, the more energy you need to expend when you physically exert yourself. The vitality facts: you need to build muscle and improve the efficiency of your cardio-vascular system.*

*Read about these energy-sappers and kick them out of your life! Then try out fatigue-fighters to rev up your system and put you into first gear...*

**Eating for energy:** *Low-fat proteins, such as chicken and fish, fire your energy and are top choices for lunch. Over-eating and eating heavy meals can make you feel sluggish. Don't eat later than 8 pm if you can avoid it.*

*Choose foods that fuel your system with sustained energy, rather than the quick highs and subsequent lows of refined carbohydrates. If you get hungry between meals, have nutritious* snacks such as sugar-free fruit and nut bars, carob instead of chocolate, crudités and raw fruit.

**Drink lots of water during the day:** *Dehydration can slow you up. If you feel drained, drink a glass of water with a 1 g tablet (dissolved) of vitamin C.*

**Flex your mental muscle:** *Just as you have to find a sport or regime which works for you, so you must develop a personal working style to release your mental energy. Get to know your own span of concentration. Even if you find it's only 10 minutes, go with that. Take a break. Don't do anything mentally distracting but use the time to, say, make a drink. It will work like the 'exercise-rest-exercise' pattern recommended by physical energy experts. Just as muscles repair and strengthen while you rest, so the work you leave will register and consolidate in your mind, and you return to work refreshed.*

**Inject some fun and variety into your routine with a new pastime, a fresh challenge.**

## SPA CLEANSING DIET

Escape to a spa or health farm for a few days and you'll discover that the beauty treatments, fresh, nutritious foods and extra rest will leave you de-stressed and revitalized.

At the sparkling blue and white Biotherm Thalassotherapy Centre, built at the sea's edge in historic Deauville, in north-west France, sea-water and seaweed treatments tone your body from the outside, while unique dietetic meals nourish and cleanse your system from the inside.

Create a mini-spa at home one weekend: treat yourself to a facial, body scrub, and pedicure. Increase your oxygen intake with lots of walking, cycling, riding or other sports. And follow the principles of the Biotherm eating plan for two days.

**Drink 2 litres ($3\frac{1}{2}$–4 pints) liquid per day,** made up of 50% lightly mineralized water and 50% fruit juices or tisanes.

**Recommended tisanes** Burdock, for its blood purifying properties; menthol, a liver regulator; ginseng, sage and rosemary, for their properties as tonics.

**Breakfast** Cereal with skimmed milk, natural yogurt and a fruit cocktail of apricots and peaches. Plus a boiled egg for protein.

**Lunchtime** Steamed fish and a salad of raw carrots, cucumber, tomatoes.

**Afternoon** Enjoy another fruit cocktail of apricots, peaches and oranges.

**Early evening** Make a carrot or tomato soup, followed by chicken with lightly steamed vegetables.

# index

**173**

# Acknowledgements

**Chrissie Painell** would like to thank the following for their assistance in the production of this book: *Eve Cameron, Susan Chance, Pat Ingram, Fiona MacIntyre, Sarita Montrose, Esme Newton-Dunn, Frank Phillips, Lisa Podmore.*

### Credits

Sunglasses, pg 81, by Alain Mikli; Perfume bottle, pg 112 by Annick Goutal from Les Senteurs, Ebury Street SW1; Watch, pg 84 The Watch Gallery, Fulham Road SW3. The healthy cocktails featured on pg 60–61 were supplied by: Coconut Grove; The Cocktail Shop; Barts's wholefood restaurant, Ashtead, Surrey; Christy's vegetarian restaurant.

Cover photograph: by Tony McGee. Styling by Mark Connolly. Hair by Sally Francomb for Vincent Lonnro. Make-up by Leanne Hirsh at Lynne Franks. Jacket, skirt, hat by Betty Jackson. Leggings, shoes, belt by Pineapple. Gloves by Dents.

Jacket photograph: Russ Malkin

### Photographic Credits

pg 14 Richard Haughton; pg 22 Bugzester; pg 22 Robert Erdmann; pg 27 Camera Press; pg 27 P Demarchelier/Marie Claire, pg 35 Nick D'Alessio; pg 39 Rau Wolf/Marie Claire; pg 43 Nabon; pg 47 Richard Dunkley; pg 51 Perlstein/Transworld; pg 55 Perlstein/Transworld; pg 59 Perlstein/Transworld; pg 63 Perlstein/Transworld; pg 67 Robert Erdmann; pg 71 All Sport; pg 75 Anna/Transworld; pg 79 Costantino Ruspoli; pg 83 Robert Erdmann; pg 87 Robert Erdmann; pg 90–91 Robert Erdmann; pg 91 Robert Erdmann; pg 95 Moser/Marie Claire; pg 103 Costantino Ruspoli; pg 111 Camera Press; pg 114 Graham Peebles; pg 118 Gan/Transworld; pg 131 Nick D'Alessio; pg 139 Ariel Skelley; pg 143 Skishoot; pg 146–147 Bugzester; pg 154/ Grazia/Transworld; pg 154/5 Sandra Lousada; pg 159 Bialas; pg 162–3 Nick D'Alessio; pg 167 Denis Boussard.